DEBATABLE TOPICS IN PCOS PATIENTS

Edited by **Neeraj Kumar Agrawal** and **Kiran Singh**

Debatable Topics in PCOS Patients

http://dx.doi.org/10.5772/intechopen.68300
Edited by Neeraj Kumar Agrawal and Kiran Singh

Contributors

Elham Pourmatroud, Nyengidiki Kennedy Tamunomie, Vadeneme Oriji, Wen-Long Hu, Yen-Nung Liao, Yu-Chiang Hung, Mojca Jensterle, Simona Ferjan, Andrej Janez, Filiz Cebeci, Işık Kaban, Melek Aslan Kayıran, Vefa Asli Erdemir, Cringu Antoniu Ionescu, Ina Popescu, Mihai Banacu, Mihai Dimitriu, N.K. Agrawal

Published by InTech
Janeza Trdine 9, 51000 Rijeka, Croatia

Publishing Process Manager Maja Bozicevic
Technical Editor SPi Global
Cover InTech Design team

First published February, 2018
Printed in Croatia
Legal deposit, Croatia: National and University Library in Zagreb

Additional hard copies can be obtained from orders@intechopen.com

Debatable Topics in PCOS Patients, Edited by Neeraj Kumar Agrawal and Kiran Singh
p. cm.
Print ISBN 978-953-51-3811-2
Online ISBN 978-953-51-3812-9

For EU product safety concerns:
IN TECH d.o.o., Prolaz Marije Krucifikse Kozulić 3, 51000 Rijeka, Croatia,
info@intechopen.com or visit our website at intechopen.com.

Meet the editor

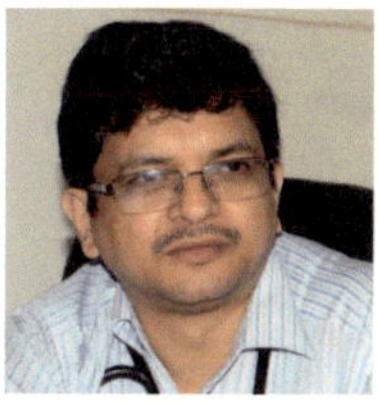

Prof. Neeraj Kumar Agrawal, DM (Endocrinology), is Professor and the Head of the Department of Endocrinology and Metabolism, Institute of Medical Sciences, Banaras Hindu University, Varanasi, India. He has clinical and research training in endocrinology and metabolism. He completed his DM course in 2000 and since then is actively involved in teaching and training in the subspeciality. He has keen interest in reproductive endocrinology and adolescent endocrinology, diabetes and thyroid disorders. He has published over 80 scientific publications in peer-reviewed journals and conference proceedings. He has edited a book on "Thyroid Hormone". He is an examiner to training centres of endocrinology. He is actively involved in the Endocrine Society of India and is a speaker in annual conferences.

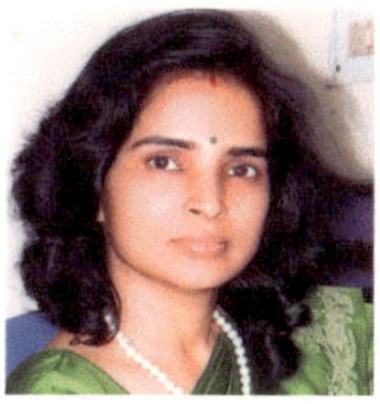

Kiran Singh, PhD, is an Assistant Professor in the Department of Molecular and Human Genetics, Banaras Hindu University, Varanasi, India. She completed her PhD degree in the year 2005 from Cytogenetic Laboratory, Banaras Hindu University, Varanasi, India. She specializes in reproductive genetics including diabetes and diabetic foot ulcer genetics, genetics of male and female infertility, PCOS, endometriosis and recurrent miscarriage. She has over 65 scientific publications in peer-reviewed national and international journals with good citations. She is a principal or key investigator on over eight active grants. She has also published a book on male infertility under Springer publication and many book chapters. She has many recognitions and awards to her credit. She is an editorial member and academic editor of many reputed journals. She has also delivered invited lectures in national and international conferences.

Contents

Preface

Polycystic ovarian syndrome affects females in reproductive age and may affect up to late reproductive life. The disease produces considerable morbidity, and one of its foremost phenotypes, hirsutism, produces considerable psychological stress in women. Its clinical features are widely variable and are not solely diagnostic of polycystic ovarian disease. The definitions of the disease remains elusive. This can be deciphered from the several diagnostic criteria put forward by different societies from time to time. Various definitions have tried to take into account the pathophysiology of the disease, but the final word is not yet out. The controversy continues whether gonadotropin levels or polycystic morphology of the ovary is the diagnostic abnormality. Polycystic ovarian syndrome is a disorder of excess androgen, primary or secondary to multiple aetiologies. There are metabolic changes involving carbohydrate and fat metabolism and increased cardiovascular risk and fatalities. Large numbers of patients are relieved of the problem, while many of them are still perplexed as the disease rages unabated.

For clinicians and researchers alike, polycystic ovarian syndrome is currently an intriguing entity. The controversy on the primary etiological factors and organ of origin of the disorder is persisting. The genetic and environmental factors interplay and produce a spectrum of the disorder. Obesity plays a crucial role in the clinical picture. Hirsutism resolves in many but may be problematic in some patients. Lifestyle changes are sheet anchor, but hormonal control poses challenges to clinician. The treatment is mostly unsatisfactory. The modifiable factors in patients must be consistently addressed for improving the outcome from metabolic and cardiovascular complications.

The book has been written keeping in mind the controversies of definition, pathophysiology and clinical implications of the disease and tries to put forth the available literature. The discussion will improve understanding of the disease process and help the readers to care for patients at large.

Prof. Neeraj Kumar Agrawal
Professor and Head
Department of Endocrinology and Metabolism
Institute of Medical Sciences, Banaras Hindu University
Varanasi, India

Dr. Kiran Singh
Assistant Professor
Department of Molecular and Human Genetics
Institute of Science, Banaras Hindu University
Varanasi, India

Section 1

Introduction

Chapter 1

Introductory Chapter: Polycystic Ovarian Disease: The Rainbow Without Color (SPECTRUM)

Abha Kiran, Uma Pandey and
Neeraj Kumar Agarwal

Additional information is available at the end of the chapter

http://dx.doi.org/10.5772/intechopen.73335

1. Introduction

The term polycystic ovarian disease is a misnomer. The question whether it is a disease whole by itself or a sign of a wider disease complex has eluded many physicians from early 1900s. The insult to the normal physiology occurs in adolescence or the cause is deep rooted during the genesis of life; that is, fertilization and embryo formation are not clear yet. It is said that a person diagnosed with polycystic ovarian disease in adulthood can have signs and symptoms of metabolic syndrome in future. It is one disease that affects an young girl who is being bullied for her hairy faces, and blisters on her faces to a women who is trying hard to work with her irregular and scanty periods, to women hoping to become pregnant and have a baby and to a middle aged women who has to remember to take her daily dosage of antihypertensive medication. With increasing number of patients presenting with symptoms of polycystic ovarian disease, the day is not far when it will become an emerging medical challenge.

2. The challenges in diagnosis

There has been long debate regarding the definition and diagnostic criteria of polycystic ovarian disease. The diagnostic criteria can be dated back to 1990, when National Institute of Child Health and Human Development (NICHD) gave the first working diagnostic criteria [1].The NICHD criteria was based on majority opinion and was not on clinical trial [2]. Polycystic morphology of the ovaries was a consistent finding in women demonstrating biochemical and clinical evidence of the syndrome [3–6] that was not included in NICHD criteria. Then came the guideline by European Society for Reproduction and Embryology (ESHRE) and the American society for Reproductive Medicine (ASRM) criteria in 2003, which included the ultrasonographic finding of polycystic ovaries. The Rotterdam criteria are controversial.

Fulfilling two of three diagnostic criteria implies that PCOS can be diagnosed in the absence of androgen excess or menstrual irregularity—the very factors that were once considered absolute requisite for the syndrome [7]. Task force appointed by the Androgen Excess and PCOS society in 2006 considered the menstrual disorder and the ultrasonography finding of polycystic ovaries to be the presentation of similar pathophysiology and considered them to be one. At present, there is no definitive diagnostic criteria for polycystic ovarian disease rather it is a diagnosis of exclusion [7]. For evaluation of hyperandrogenemia, there is no consensus about which testosterone to be measured, when to be measured, what range should be taken, and what method of measurement is to be used. For features of hyperandrogenism assessment of hirsutism, acne and alopecia are more of subjective feature. Assessment of menstrual irregularities and serum progesterone for anovulation is also not confirmatory. Ultrasonographic findings of polycystic ovary are also subjective. None of the above criteria states for diagnosis of polycystic disease in adolescents where these features could be present due to pubertal changes [8–10].

3. The challenges for pathophysiological basis

There has been extensive work on finding the etiology and pathophysiology behind this disease. None could find exact etiology behind this. There is halt in the dynamic endocrinal milieu of the ovary [1]. There is increase in both LH pulse frequency and production of more bioactive LH, and there is increased LH:FSH ratio leading to neuroendocrinologic origin hypothesis. The feedback signal from periphery may be inappropriate or there may be intrinsic hypothalamic dysfunction [1]. Hyperandrogenemia came into scene while searching for a cause of both aberrant peripheral feedback and dysfunctional hypothalamus. The rises in androgen were both from ovary and adrenal glands, shifting the focus on ovarian pathology [11–14]. Some attribute the chronic anovulation to be the cause of hyperandrogenemia, and some authors say the other way. Insulin resistance causes hyperandrogenemia. Insulin causes selective stimulation of receptor that causes hyperandrogenemia. About 35% of patients have impaired glucose tolerance and 7–10% have diabetes mellitus [1]. It is a more common finding in obese polycystic disease patient than in lean PCOS patient. Nearly 25–50% of women with PCOS have no demonstrable insulin resistance. Approximately 60% of women with PCOS are obese. The prevalence of PCOS is comparable in women with BMI <18.5, normal weight women, and BMI 25–30 and BMI ≥ 30 [1]. Modern lifestyle and obesity can also be the cause. Recent researchers are giving significance to the genetic cause. There are genetic and nongenetic theories for etiopathogenesis of polycystic ovarian disease. Recently, two-hit hypothesis has been given. Patient presenting with PCOS are thought be genetically predisposed, and after environmental insult, they become symptomatic. Genetic predisposition can be because of mutations affecting ovarian function, female virilization, or intrauterine nutritional status of fetus. Environmental insult can be hyperinsulinemia, obesity, and others. There has been evolutionary theory behind PCOS; to compensate for hyperandrogenemia in male, there was evolutionary decrease in female fertility and also that in the process of evolution a more androgenic environment helped nutritionally deprived population to reproduce which in today's scenario is not beneficial [11].

4. The challenges in treatment and outcome

As cause and pathophysiology is not clear, the treatment ranges widely from only lifestyle modification to planned use of insulin sensitizers like metformin to desperate ovarian drilling, there is also indecisiveness about the usefulness of present treatment methods in ameliorating long-term complications like endometrial carcinoma. A simple initial step of losing weight can return ovulation in patients. Losing weight alone does not cure other symptoms. For menstrual irregularity, continuous or cyclical hormonal therapy can be used. For infertility treatment, simple weight loss can return ovulation or patients have many time opt for in-vitro fertilization. Metformin as primary drug for ovulation is controversial though it improves insulin-resistant status.

The determinants for calculating the prognosis of the patient are also not clear. With different age of population presenting with different presentation and with people at increased risk for variety of problems like infertility, dysfunctional bleeding, endometrial cancer, obesity, type 2 diabetes mellitus, dyslipidemia, hypertension, and cardiovascular disease, it is difficult to frame a prognostic criteria.

Author details

Abha Kiran[1], Uma Pandey[1]* and Neeraj Kumar Agarwal[2]

*Address all correspondence to: uma.pandey2006@yahoo.com

1 Department of Obstetrics and Gynaecology, Institute of Medical Sciences, Banaras Hindu University, Varanasi, India

2 Department of Endocrinology, Institute of Medical Sciences, Banaras Hindu University, Varanasi, India

References

[1] Speroff L, Fritz MA. Chapter 12, Chronic anovulation and the polycystic ovary syndrome. In: Clinical Gynecologic Endocrinology and Infertility. 8th ed. Philadelphia: Lippincott Williams & Wilkins; 2012. pp. 495-532

[2] Rotterdam ESHRE/ASRM-Sponsored PCOS Consensus Workshop Group. Revised 2003 consensus on diagnostic criteria and long-term health risks related to polycystic ovary syndrome. Fertility and Sterility. 2004;**81**(1):19-25

[3] Michelmore K, Ong K, Mason S, Bennett S, Perry L, Vessey M, et al. Clinical features in women with polycystic ovaries: Relationships to insulin sensitivity, insulin gene VNTR and birth weight. Clinical Endocrinology. 2001;**55**(4):439-446

[4] Carmina E, Lobo RA. Polycystic ovaries in hirsute women with normal menses. The American Journal of Medicine. 2001;**111**(8):602-606

[5] Cela E, Robertson C, Rush K, Kousta E, White DM, Wilson H, et al. Prevalence of polycystic ovaries in women with androgenic alopecia. European Journal of Endocrinology. 2003;**149**(5):439-442

[6] Cresswell J, Fraser R, Bruce C, Egger P, Phillips D, Barker DJ. Relationship between polycystic ovaries, body mass index and insulin resistance. Acta Obstetricia et Gynecologica Scandinavica. 2003;**82**(1):61-64

[7] Lujan ME, Chizen DR, Pierson RA. Diagnostic criteria for polycystic ovary syndrome: Pitfalls and controversies. Journal of Obstetrics and Gynaecology Canada. 2008 Aug;**30**(8): 671-679

[8] Roe AH, Dokras A. The diagnosis of polycystic ovary syndrome in adolescents. Reviews in Obstetrics and Gynecology. 2011;**4**(2):45-51

[9] Sultan C, Paris F. Clinical expression of polycystic ovary syndrome in adolescent girls. Fertility and Sterility. 2006;**86**(Suppl 1):S6

[10] Carmina E, Oberfield SE, Lobo RA. The diagnosis of polycystic ovary syndrome in adolescents. American Journal of Obstetrics and Gynecology. 2010;**203**:201.e1-201.e5

[11] Rosenfield RL, Ehrmann DA. The pathogenesis of polycystic ovary syndrome (PCOS): The hypothesis of PCOS as functional ovarian Hyperandrogenism revisited. Endocrine Reviews. 2016 Oct;**37**(5):467-520. Epub Jul 26, 2016

[12] Futterweit W, Deligdisch L. Histopathological effects of exogenously administered testosterone in 19 female to male transsexuals. The Journal of Clinical Endocrinology and Metabolism. 1986;**62**:16-21

[13] Goodarzi MO, Dumesic DA, Chazenbalk G, Azziz R. Polycystic ovary syndrome: Etiology, pathogenesis and diagnosis. Nature Reviews. Endocrinology. 2011 Apr;**7**(4):219-231

[14] S1 J, Eden JA. Genetic and non-genetic theories on the etiology of polycystic ovary syndrome. Gynecological Endocrinology. 1996 Oct;**10**(5):357-364

Section 2

Controversies in Pathophysiology

Chapter 2

Controversies in Polycystic Ovary Syndrome

Işık Kaban, Filiz Cebeci, Melek Aslan Kayıran and
Vefa Asli Erdemir

Additional information is available at the end of the chapter

http://dx.doi.org/10.5772/intechopen.72513

Abstract

Polycystic ovarian syndrome (PCOS) is the most common endocrinopathy that affects women from puberty to whole reproductive life. Diagnosis and treatment of PCOS is not clear. Polycystic ovary syndrome is a multisystem disease that involves dermatologist examining patients with clinical hyperandrogenism and/or biochemical signs of hyperandrogenism; gynecologist examines patients with oligo-ovulation or infertility. The management of PCOS should be tailored to each woman's specific symptoms, fertility-related implications, and metabolic disorders. Pharmacologic treatment is not necessary for all patients with PCOS, also lifestyle changes like exercise, weight loss, and diet are effective for treatment. Lifestyle changes are often recommended as first-line treatment for PCOS to benefit general health. Topical nonhormonal therapies and laser hair removal may be effective for cutaneous symptoms like acne, hirsutism, and androgenetic alopecia in the PCOS population and are useful first-line agents. Some pharmacological agents (anti-androgens) are used to control the dermatological symptoms of hyperandrogenism. Metformin is useful for metabolic and glycemic anomalies and for the treatment of menstrual irregularities, but less effective than antiandrogens for the treatment of both hirsutism and acne. The aim of this study is to talk about unclear topics in PCOS and multidisciplinary approach to patients.

Keywords: polycystic ovarian syndrome, hyperandrogenism amenorrhea, hirsutism, infertility

1. Introduction

Polycystic ovarian syndrome (PCOS) is the most common endocrine disorder among women of reproductive age but often unrecognized condition. It was first described by Stein and Leventhal in 1935 as women with polycystic ovaries, amenorrhea, and hirsutism [1]. One in

15 women worldwide is affected by this syndrome [2]. There is actually no consensus on diagnostic criteria and the figures may change.

Most women with PCOS have infertility or subfertility and other metabolic alterations such as insulin resistance, dyslipidemia, hyperinsulinemia, and obesity. Despite the etiology of the syndrome is still far from being elucidated, it could be considered the result of concurrent endocrine modifications, lifestyle factors, and genetic background. In particular, accumulating evidence suggests that insulin resistance and compensatory hyperinsulinemia play a pivotal pathogenic role in the hyperandrogenism of many PCOS phenotypes, which in turn have a clear detrimental effect on chronic anovulation [3].

There has been considerable controversy about specific diagnostic criteria when all classic features (hirsutism, irregular menstrual cycles, obesity, and a classic ovarian morphology by transvaginal ultrasonography) are not evident.

Research for PCOS in the last decade has brought new important insights for the evaluation and treatment of this disorder. Unclear points for diagnosis and treatment and proper approach to PCOS-related diseases will be discussed in this chapter.

2. Diagnosis

Some criteria have been proposed for the diagnosis of the disease but these criteria have changed several times. In fact, clinically recognized hyperandrogenism and the non-regularity of ovarian function, especially chronic anovulation, are the main criteria. Hirsutism, acne, and alopecia are clinical signs of hyperandrogenism in these women while it may be difficult to make a diagnosis due to phenotype, obesity, race/ethnicity, and environmental factors. Most of these women have polycystic ovaries that can be shown in imaging studies, but this is not a criterion for diagnosis because many healthy women may have polycystic ovaries. The diagnosis of the polycystic ovary was also revised. Most of the researchers used the presence of at least 12 follicles (measuring 2–9 mm in diameter) in each ovarian as a criterion prior to 2014. Dewailly et al. reported that the threshold value of ≥25 follicles is significant for diagnosis [4]. In addition, it is not uncommon for PCOS to coexist with obesity, insulin resistance, dyslipidemia, endothelial dysfunction, and other metabolic disorders. All of these suggests metabolic syndrome.

2.1. Diagnostic criteria

According to 1990 National Institutes of Health (NIH) criteria, hyperandrogenemia findings and ovulation disorder were defined as PCOS. In 2003, Rotterdam criteria for PCOS diagnosis were accepted by the NIH (**Table 1**) [5].

General agreement exists among specialty society guidelines that the diagnosis of PCOS must be based on the presence of at least two of the following three criteria: chronic anovulation, hyperandrogenism (clinical or biological), and polycystic ovaries [6].

http://dx.doi.org/10.5772/intechopen.72513

	NIH 1990 criteria	Rotterdam criteria [5]	AE-PCOS Society criteria
Hyperandrogenism	Required	Two of three required	Required
Ovulatory dysfunction (oligo- or amenorrhea)	Required	Two of three required	Either ovulatory dysfunction or PCOS morphology required
PCOS morphology	Not required	Two of three required	Either ovulatory dysfunction or PCOS morphology required

Table 1. Diagnostic criteria for PCOS.

2.1.1. *Detecting of ovulatory dysfunction*

The definition of ovulatory dysfunction is not clear. If the menstrual cycle length is longer than 35 days, it is assumed that chronic anovulation is present and that special tests are not needed. A 30–35 day cycle can also be anovulatory. Measurement of serum progesterone in the mid-luteal stage (Days 21–22) is the best way to evaluate ovulation. Progesterone levels > 2.5 ng/mL may indicate ovulation but values of ≥7 ng/mL are needed for normal luteal function [7]. Three consecutive measurements with a total serum value of ≥15 ng/mL indicate normal luteal function. Alternatives to progesterone measurement such as baseline body temperature schedules, urinary luteinizing hormone (LH) kits, or timed endometrial biopsy may be suggested, but do not provide sufficient information about the luteal phase. The cycle time for oligomenorrhea is ≥35 days in adult women. The threshold value during puberty is higher and a cycle length of up to 40 days can be considered normal.

2.1.2. *Measurement of androgens*

In women, the androgen source is the adrenal cortex and the ovaries. Testosterone is produced from the ovary, DHEA-S is produced from the adrenal gland, and androstenedione is produced from both adrenal and ovarian.

The issue of which serum androgen should be measured for diagnosis of PCOS remains controversial. Free testosterone (T) levels are more sensitive than the measurement of total T for establishing the existence of androgen excess. The normal value of total testosterone level is 20–60 ng/dl. In cases with PCOS, the total testosterone level is generally lower than 150 ng/dl. If the total testosterone level is higher than 150 ng/dl, testosterone-secreting adrenal tumor, ovarian tumor, or ovarian hypertrophy should be suspected. In patients using oral contraceptives, total androgen levels should be measured 8–12 weeks after drug withdrawal.

Direct analog RIA measurement in commercial laboratories is notoriously inaccurate. Ideally, it should be determined through equilibrium dialysis techniques. Consequently, if the clinician is uncertain regarding the quality of the free-T assay, it may be preferable to rely on calculated free T, which has a good concordance and correlation with free T as measured by equilibrium dialysis methods [8]. Value of measuring levels of androgens other than T (dehydroepiandrosterone sulfate, androstenedione) in patients with PCOS is relatively insignificant. If dehydroepiandrostenedione sulfate (DHEAS) levels are higher than 700 μg/dL, adrenal tumors should be suspected. DHEAS levels may also increase in cases with LOCAH (late-onset congenital adrenal hyperplasia), Cushing's disease, adrenal adenomas as well as PCOS.

2.2. Other laboratory tests

Patients with non-classical 21-hydroxylase deficiency may develop as PCOS hyperandrogenism, anovulation, and PCO. Therefore, evaluation of serum 17 hydroxyprogesterone (17OH-PG) should be always included in a diagnostic study [9, 10]. Serum 17OH-PG levels higher than 10 ng/mL indicates the presence of 21-hydroxylase deficiency, while values between 2 and 10 ng/mL suggest that further testing with adrenocorticotropic hormone stimulation is needed [10]. Serum AMH > 5 ng/mL is also reported to be significant for PCOS [11].

2.2.1. Evaluation of ovarian morphology

Ovarian morphology is usually evaluated by transvaginal ultrasonography. Transabdominal ultrasonography may be used for virgin patients, but ovarian morphology assessment and especially the calculation of the number of small follicles may be difficult. Ultrasonographic imaging technology has been rapidly developing and the clinician should know that the number of follicles visible is related to ultrasound quality [4]. According to current Rotterdam guidelines, PCO is defined as the presence of at least 12 follicles measured 2–9 mm or an increased ovarian size (>10 mL) (**Figure 1**) [12]. The new AES guidelines, based on the observation of published data using new ultrasound technology, increased the threshold number of small ovarian follicles to 25 [4]. The ovarian size threshold is unaffected by new technologies and the threshold between normal and increased ovarian size is assumed to be 10 mL. In some populations, during puberty or aging, a different threshold for ovarian size may be suggested [13].

2.2.2. Clinical signs of hyperandrogenism

Hirsutism is defined as excessive hair growth in women in a manner consistent with androgen sensitivity. Typically, hirsutism in PCOS is followed by initial menarche, whereas in some of the adolescent girls, pubic hair development and hirsutism had already begun 25–33% of white women have terminal hair on the upper lip, periareolar area or linea-alba, but hirsutism and various other hyperandrogenic disorders are more prominent in PCOS. The presence of substantial numbers of terminal hairs over the chin, neck, lower face, and sideburns (particularly if extending medially) indicates the presence of androgen excess. It should be noted that ethnic differences in the number of hair follicles present and individual skin sensitivity of the

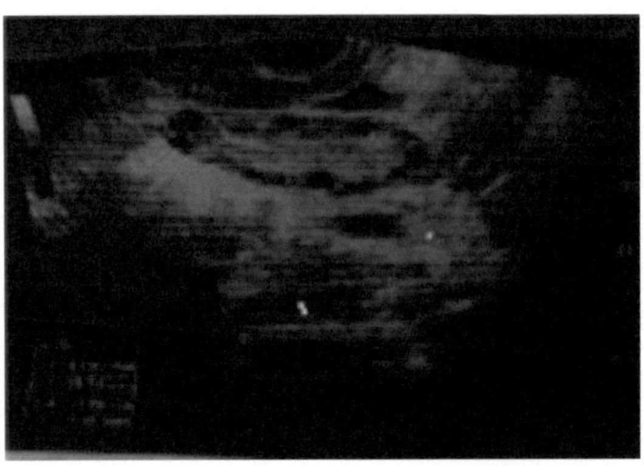

Figure 1. Transvaginal sonographic view of a polycystic ovary syndrome patient (Işık Kaban M.D. photo archive).

pilosebaceous unit to androgens are major determinants of the presence of hirsutism, as well as acne and androgenic alopecia (**Figures 2–5**) [14]. Ferriman-Gallwey scale has been the most widely used for evaluating hirsutism, but it is limited by its subjective nature and failure to include the sideburn, perineal, or buttock areas [15]. In this system, nine regions in the body are

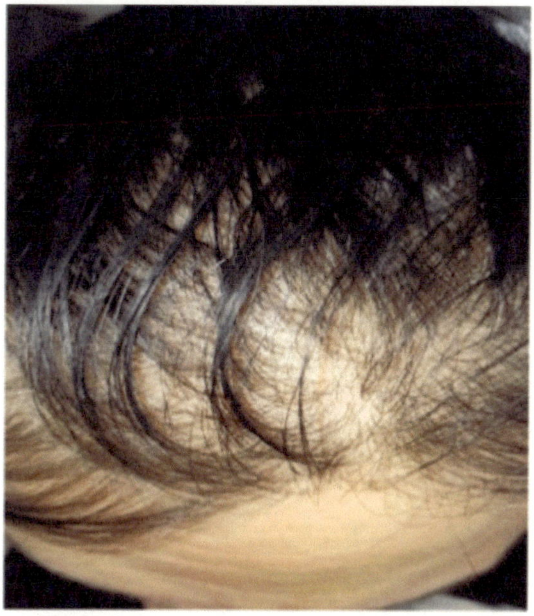

Figure 2. Androgenetic alopecia.

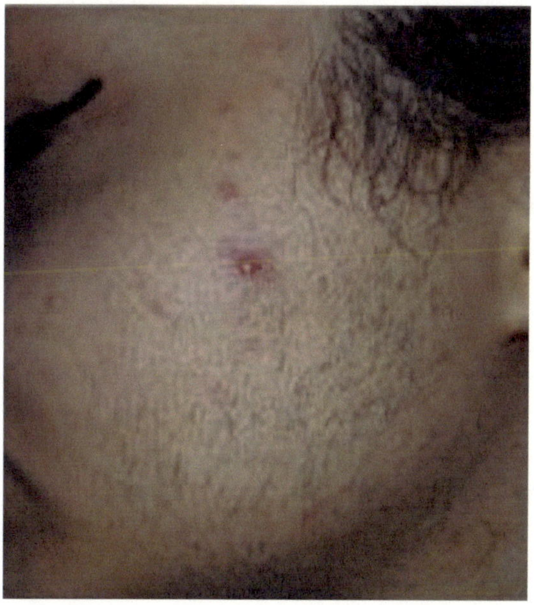

Figure 3. Acne and facial hirsutism.

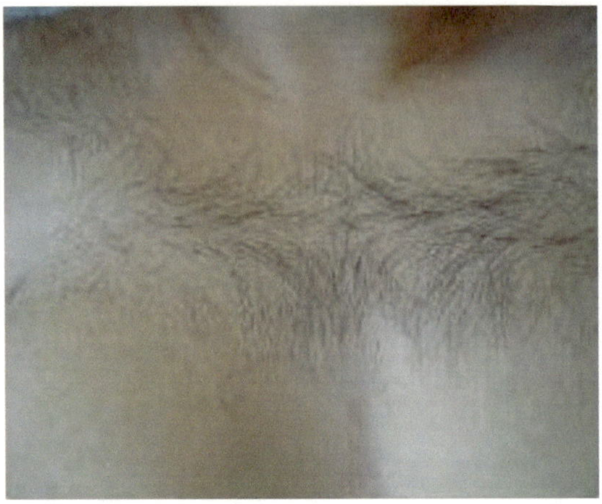

Figure 4. Hirsutism.

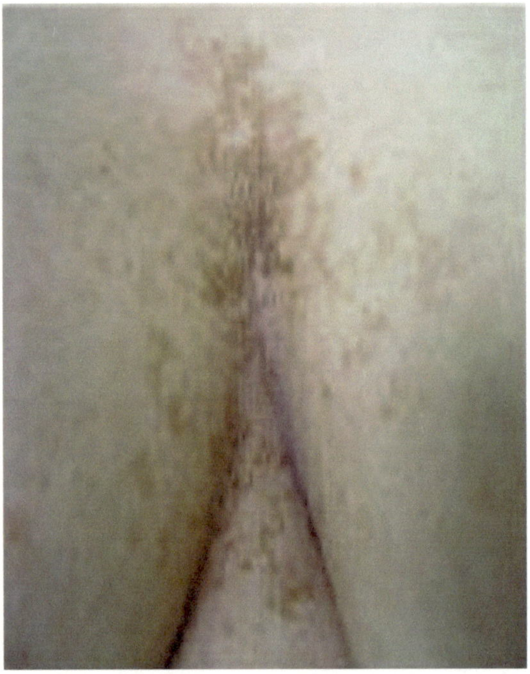

Figure 5. Acanthosis nigricans.

scaled from zero (no terminal hair) to four (excess hair). Above eight is regarded as hirsutism. Additionally, acne, androgenetic alopecia, and virilization indications (clitoromegaly, muscle mass increase, voice thickening, diminution of breast size, libido increase) should be examined.

Ferriman-Gallwey scoring system for hirsutism: upper lip, chin, chest, upper back, lower back, upper abdomen, upper arm, forearm, and thigh/leg are the body parts used for hirsutism diagnosis.

At this point, the differential diagnosis of these patients is important. Late-onset congenital adrenal hyperplasia (LOCAH) should be remembered especially in puberty patients. The use of drugs such as methyltestosterone, anabolic steroids (norethandrolone, etc.), phenytoin, diazoxide, danazol, cyclosporin, valproic acid, and minoxidil, which stimulate hair growth with androgenic effect, should be questioned. In terms of Cushing's disease, findings such as stria, central obesity, buffalo hump, and plethora should be investigated. Galactore should be investigated for hyperprolactinemia.

Acne is another clinical sign of hyperandrogenism. The likelihood of developing PCOS in girls with severe acne or acne resistant to treatment may be up to 40% in adolescents [16, 17]. In cases with persisting after adolescence, or aggravating by mid-20s, hyperandrogenemia is common and acne can be considered a clinical sign of hyperandrogenism. However, during adolescence, acne should not be considered a substitute for hyperandrogenism [18].

Only those with acne can have serum free T levels as well as those seen in hyperandrogenic disease states. Likewise, hirsutism without acne is also the case [17].

Hair loss in women with hyperandrogenism is variable. Women with severe hyperandrogenemia may experience bitemporal hair loss and loss of the frontal hairline [19].

2.2.3. *Treatment options for women with hyperandrogenism*

Some pharmacological agents (anti-androgens) are used to control the dermatological symptoms of hyperandrogenism. Oral contraceptive agents can effectively reduce the androgenic effect by increasing the sexual hormone binding globulin and/or suppressing ovarian production of androgens. In addition, physiologic doses of dexamethasone or prednisone may directly reduce adrenal androgen production. The basic mechanism of anti-androgen therapy is competitive antagonism of the androgen receptor or inhibition of 5α-reductase to prevent the conversion of testosterone to its more potent form, 5α-dihydrotestosterone. Spironolactone, cyproterone acetate, and flutamide are effective with competitive antagonism and finasteride is effective with the inhibition of 5α-reductase.

The mainstay of primary care is oral contraceptive therapy for dermatological problems in hyperandrogenism. Oral contraceptives contain estrogen (ethinyl estradiol) and a progestin. A 20–35 μg of daily ethinyl estradiol effectively suppresses pituitary-ovarian axis and reduces ovarian androgen production. The ideal progestin to be used in PCOS is progestins with the lowest androgenic profile such as chloramidon and drospirenone; however, these may induce venous thrombosis and are contraindicated in obese patients. Oral contraceptives induce the synthesis of sex hormone binding protein (SHBP) from the liver and may be more effective in controlling hirsutism and acne than transdermal or vaginal ring preparations. These formulations may be combined with anti-androgenic therapy to achieve a better response against hirsutism. Spironolactone is an aldosterone antagonist and widely used androgen blocker, its progestational activity may also reduce levels of the gonadotropin-releasing hormone. Spironolactone can induce hyperkalemia. Headaches and dizziness as side effects are relatively frequent, and the patient should increase water and salt intake during hot weather. Spironolactone can cause intermenstrual spotting in about half of women.

Finasteride is a 5α-reductase inhibitor and may decrease DHT levels by 50–60%. Significant anti-androgenic effects were shown after 6 months of treatment at 5 mg/day dose [20, 21]. The use of 5α-reductase inhibition therapy should be considered when the previous therapy with oral contraceptive and spironolactone is relatively ineffective [22]. Dutasteride, another anti-androgen molecule which has limited data, reduces plasma DHT more significantly than finasteride and inhibits the conversion of testosterone to dihydrotestosterone by the inhibition of 5α-reductase isoenzymes [23].

Metformin is an alternative therapy for hirsutism in women with PCOS who have other indications for the use of metformin. This oral antidiabetic drug is useful for metabolic and glycemic anomalies and for the treatment of menstrual irregularities, but less effective than antiandrogens for the treatment of both hirsutism and acne [22, 24].

It should be remembered that hirsutism treatment is a continuing treatment that the medical treatment response does not occur 6 months before the hair cycle and individualization of the treatment are necessary.

2.3. PCOS in the adolescent

PCOS commonly presents in the adolescence; underestimation may be more in this period because of some confounding factors such as acne, menstrual irregularities, and hirsutism [25]. These factors may also be observed in normal puberty thus misdiagnosis may be common. Anovulatory cycles and menstrual irregularities with variable cycle length are common during first years following menarche due to the immaturity of the hypothalamic-pituitary-ovarian axis. Additionally, large, multicystic ovaries in adolescents may also be considered normal as a result of natural ovarian development. It may be acceptable to clinically follow the patient for 2–3 years in terms of defining the over dysfunction in adolescents [26].

Hyperandrogenism leading to acne and hirsutism may be associated with normal puberty rather than underlying PCOS, and hyperinsulinemia is a characteristic of normal puberty. Furthermore, ranges of laboratory values for the hyperandrogenemia and Ferriman-Gallwey scoring system are established for adults and may not be of similar clinical importance in adolescence.

On the other hand, symptoms in adolescents are heterogeneous and may change over time, PCOS diagnosis may be overlooked.

In conclusion, clinical findings for PCOS in adolescents can be confusing and laboratory measurements are important. Lower and upper bounds of testosterone are not clear in young girls [25, 27].

2.4. PCOS and malignancy

A relationship between PCOS and malignancy has been reported in the literature, but this relationship is not strong. The altered metabolic and hormonal environment among women with PCOS may increase the risk of some types of cancer.

In a systematic review by Chittenden and colleagues, they investigated the gynecological malignancy association with PCOS and reported that women with PCOS are more likely to develop endometrial cancer (odds ratio 2.70) and ovarian cancer (odds ratio 2.52) but not breast cancer [28]. John et al. compared 919 women with PCOS and 72,054 women without PCOS in their meta-analyses and reported that women of all ages with PCOS have an increased risk of endometrial cancer (odds ratio 2.79), but the risk of ovarian and breast cancer was not significantly increased overall [29]. Another meta-analysis by Holly et al. reported that the associations between PCOS and endometrial, ovarian, and breast cancer are complex [30] and argued that studies showing PCOS association with endometrial cancer do not take into account body mass index (BMI) criteria. BMI is a strong and well-established risk factor for endometrial cancer. In these women, the oligomenorrheic environment increases hyperplasia and cancer risk. Prevention of oligomenorrhea by providing cyclic progesterone supplementation is important for reducing risk [31].

As a result, the risk of endometrial cancer in women with PCOS may be increased [32]. However, there is no clear association between other types of cancer and PCOS.

3. Dermatological approach to polycystic ovarian syndrome

Polycystic ovary syndrome is a multisystem disease that involves dermatologist examining patients with clinical hyperandrogenism and/or biochemical signs of hyperandrogenism; gynecologist examines patients with oligo-ovulation or infertility.

Although PCOS is a heterogeneous disorder without an easily identified single etiology, the key pathophysiologic components appear to include androgen excess, abnormal gonadotropin dynamics, and insulin resistance. Patients should be informed about long-term treatment, including lifestyle changes with systemic treatment. Success in effective management of women with PCOS is a synchronized effort between dermatologist, endocrinologist, obstetrician, nutritionist, and physical trainer [33].

4. Treatment

Lifestyle changes, local treatment approaches, and pharmacological treatment will review under the heading of treatment.

In cases with PCOS, lifestyle modification resulting from medical nutrition therapy and exercise is effective in improving clinical signs and symptoms of hyperandrogenemia. With lifestyle changes, SHBG levels increase as serum androgen levels decrease as a result of weight loss. Stop smoking is also important to reduce the complications of oral contraceptive use [33].

Local treatment; hair removal methods such as hair bleaching, tearing, shaving, waxing, electrolysis, laser hair removal, and local drug application such as eflornithine are used. It can be applied as a single treatment in the case of localized small incisions. Medical treatment is applied when waiting for the response. It has been shown that shaving does not increase the formation of new hair, and it should be explained that the illness should not underestimate this concern. It has been shown that laser epilation can treat up to 2 years hirsutism in randomized controlled trials. Since hair follicle stimulation continues in hyperandrogenic women, hair growth after laser epilation repeats. About 13.9% eflornithine topical cream inhibits DNA synthesis by inhibiting ornithine decarboxylase enzyme and suppresses the mitotic activity of the hair follicle. Terminal hair growth begins again when the drug is stopped.

Patients with polycystic ovarian syndrome are referred to clinics of dermatology with cutaneous androgenesis findings such as hirsutism, acne, and alopecia. For this reason, pharmacological treatment is often required to treat hyperandrogenemia. It should be remembered that hirsutism treatment is a continuing treatment, which the medical treatment response does not occur 6 months before the hair cycle and individualization of the treatment is necessary. Treatment may not be necessary for the patients who do not worry about hirsutism, planning to be pregnant, and regular menstrual cycles. OCSs are used as the only medication in mild hirsutism cases, while OCSs are used in combination with other antiandrogen drugs in severe and moderate hirsutism. Hirsutism adolescent girls respond perfectly to medical treatment. The combination of spironolactone and an oral contraceptive provides effective medical treatment. This combination also improves spironolactone-related menstrual irregularities. If there is no response after 6 months of treatment, the treatment should be changed. The combination of mechanical and medical treatment provides a rapid and effective remedy. The average duration of treatment is 2–3 years. Because the underlying cause is persistent, local or drug treatment does not completely cease, and the complaints start again after the treatment is discontinued.

Insulin-sensitizing drugs (metformin and pioglitazone) are used in the treatment of hyperandrogenemic patients with severe insulin resistance syndrome. It should not be used as a primary treatment in incontinent cases. Metformin is preferred for patients with PCOS with glucose intolerance. In these cases, metformin may contribute to other treatments on hirsutism. Glitazones are not recommended for treatment of hirsutism due to possible cardiovascular side effects. It is the first choice in the treatment of menstrual and ovulatory dysfunction, especially in obese cases of lifestyle change and weight loss.

Author details

Işık Kaban[1*], Filiz Cebeci[2], Melek Aslan Kayıran[2] and Vefa Asli Erdemir[2]

*Address all correspondence to: drisik@mynet.com

1 Istanbul Education and Research Hospital, Istanbul, Turkey

2 Medeniyet University Göztepe Education and Research Hospital, Istanbul, Turkey

References

[1] Stein IF, Leventhal. Amenorrhoea associated with bilateral polycystic ovaries. American Journal of Obstetrics and Gynecology. 1935;**29**:181-191

[2] Norman RJ, Dewailly D, Legro RS, Hickey TE. Polycystic ovary syndrome. Lancet (London, England). 2007;**370**(9588):685-697

[3] Chiofalo B, Laganà AS, Palmara V, Granese R, Corrado G, Mancini E, Triolo O, Ban Frangež H, Vrtačnik-Bokal E. Fasting as possible complementary approach for polycystic ovary syndrome: Hope or hype? Medical Hypotheses. 2017;**105**:1-3

[4] Dewailly D et al. Definition and significance of polycystic ovarian morphology: A task force report from the androgen excess and polycystic ovary syndrome society. Human Reproduction Update. 2014;**20**(3):334-352

[5] The Rotterdam ESHRE/ASRM-Sponsored PCOS Consensus Workshop Group. Revised 2003 consensus on diagnostic criteria and long-term health risks related to polycystic ovary syndrome (PCOS). Human Reproduction. 2004;**19**(1):41-47

[6] Goodman NF, Cobin RH, Futterweit W, Glueck JS, Legro RS, Carmina E. American Association of Clinical Endocrinologists, American College of Endocrinology, and androgen excess and PCOS society disease state clinical review: Guide to the best practices in the evaluation and treatment of polycystic ovary syndrome-part 1. Endocrine Practice. 2016;**21**(11):1291-1300

[7] Hull MG, Savage PE, Bromham DR, Ismail AA, Morris AF. The value of a single serum progesterone measurement in the midluteal phase as a criterion of a potentially fertile cycle ('ovulation') derived form treated and untreated conception cycles. Fertility and Sterility. 1982;**37**(3):355-360

[8] Vermeulen A, Verdonck L, Kaufman JM. A critical evaluation of simple methods for the estimation of free testosterone in serum. The Journal of Clinical Endocrinology and Metabolism. 1999;**84**(10):3666-3672

[9] Franks S. The investigation and management of hirsutism. The Journal of Family Planning and Reproductive Health Care. 2012;**38**(3):182-186

[10] Carmina E. Hirsutism: Investigation and management. Expert Review of Endocrinology and Metabolism. 2010;**5**(2):189-195

[11] Dewailly D et al. Diagnosis of polycystic ovary syndrome (PCOS): Revisiting the threshold values of follicle count on ultrasound and of the serum AMH level for the definition of polycystic ovaries. Human Reproduction. 2011;**26**(11):3123-3129

[12] Balen AH, Laven JSE, Tan SL, Dewailly D. Ultrasound assessment of the polycystic ovary: International consensus definitions. Human Reproduction Update. 2003;**9**(6):505-514

[13] Chen Y et al. Ovarian volume and follicle number in the diagnosis of polycystic ovary syndrome in Chinese women. Ultrasound in Obstetrics & Gynecology. 2008;**32**(5):700-703

[14] Rosenfield RL, Deplewski D. Role of androgens in the developmental biology of the pilosebaceous unit. The American Journal of Medicine. 1995;**98**(1 SUPPL. 1)

[15] Hatch R, Rosenfield RL, Kim MH, Tredway D. Current developments hirsutism: Implications, etiology, and management. American Journal of Obstetrics and Gynecology. 1981;**140**:815-830

[16] Timpatanapong P, Rojanasakul A. Hormonal profiles and prevalence of polycystic ovary syndrome in women with acne. The Journal of Dermatology. 1997;**24**(4):223-229

[17] Lucky AW, McGuire J, Rosenfield RL, Lucky PA, Rich BH. Plasma androgens in women with acne vulgaris. The Journal of Investigative Dermatology. 1983;**81**(1):70-74

[18] Roe AH, Dokras A. The diagnosis of polycystic ovary syndrome in adolescents. Reviews in Obstetrics & Gynecology. 2011;**4**(2):45-51

[19] Carmina E, Lobo RA. Treatment of hyperandrogenic alopecia in women. Fertility and Sterility. 2003;**79**(1):91-95

[20] Yeon JH et al. 5 mg/day finasteride treatment for normoandrogenic Asian women with female pattern hair loss. Journal of the European Academy of Dermatology and Venereology. 2011;**25**(2):211-214

[21] Lakryc EM, Motta ELA, Soares Jr JM, Haidar MA, de Lima GR, Baracat EC. The benefits of finasteride for hirsute women with polycystic ovary syndrome or idiopathic hirsutism. Gynecological Endocrinology. 2003;**17**(1):57-63

[22] Paparodis R, Dunaif A. The hirsute woman: Challenges in evaluation and management. Endocrine Practice. 2011;**17**(5):807-818

[23] Olszewska M, Rudnicka L. Effective treatment of female androgenic alopecia with dutasteride. Journal of Drugs in Dermatology. 2005;**4**(5):637-640

[24] Legro RS et al. Diagnosis and treatment of polycystic ovary syndrome: An Endocrine Society clinical practice guideline. The Journal of Clinical Endocrinology and Metabolism. 2013;**98**(12):4565-4592

[25] Williams RM, Ong KK, Dunger DB. Polycystic ovarian syndrome during puberty and adolescence. Molecular and Cellular Endocrinology. 2013;**373**(1-2):61-67

[26] Hardy TSE, Norman RJ. Diagnosis of adolescent polycystic ovary syndrome. Steroids. 2013;**78**(8):751-754

[27] Hickey M et al. Clinical, ultrasound and biochemical features of polycystic ovary syndrome in adolescents: Implications for diagnosis. Human Reproduction. 2011;**26**(6):1469-1477

[28] Chittenden BG, Fullerton G, Maheshwari A, Bhattacharya S. Polycystic ovary syndrome and the risk of gynaecological cancer: A systematic review. Reproductive Biomedicine Online. 2009;**19**(3):398-405

[29] Barry JA, Azizia MM, Hardiman PJ. Risk of endometrial, ovarian and breast cancer in women with polycystic ovary syndrome: A systematic review and meta-analysis. Human Reproduction Update. 2014;**20**(5):748-758

[30] Harris HR, Terry KL. Polycystic ovary syndrome and risk of endometrial, ovarian, and breast cancer: A systematic review. Fertility Research and Practice. 2016;**2**(1):14

[31] Schindler AE. Progestogen deficiency and endometrial cancer risk. Maturitas. 2009;**62**(4): 334-337

[32] Dumesic DA, Lobo RA. Cancer risk and PCOS. Steroids. 2013;**78**(8):782-785

[33] Buzney E, Sheu J, Buzney C, Reynolds RV. Polycystic ovary syndrome: A review for dermatologists: Part II. Treatment. Journal of the American Academy of Dermatology. 2014;**71**(5):859.e1-859.e15

Chapter 3

Lean Women with Polycystic Ovary Syndrome

Elham Pourmatroud

Additional information is available at the end of the chapter

http://dx.doi.org/10.5772/intechopen.70621

Abstract

Most of the time, polycystic ovary syndrome (PCOs) is considered as an obese women disease; lean PCOs patients need to evaluate and treat completely as a neglected subgroup. Androgen excess signs and symptoms, insulin resistance (IR) and its consequences, cardiometabolic risks, and regular exercise must be noted and managed carefully.

Keywords: lean, non-obese, androgen, insulin, PCO

1. Introduction

Polycystic ovary syndrome (PCOs) is the most common reason of androgen excess in reproductive-age women with a prevalence of 6.5–8% according to clinical appearance [1] or even up to 20% by sonographic evidence [2].

For the first time, Stein and Leventhal described it in the year 1935 [3]. Year after year, the description of the disease developed; in 1990, the National Institutes of Health (NIH) mentioned oligo-ovulation and hyperandrogenism with or without hyperandrogenemia (HA) must be together (of course, after exclusion of another causes of androgen excess) [4].

Another expert meeting in 2003 expanded the NIH definition of PCOs by adding the sonographic aspect of the disease (Rotterdam criteria) [5]. According to their criteria, two of three signs/symptoms are necessary for PCOs diagnosis; therefore, PCOs woman can be ovulatory with regular menstruation.

More recently, the Androgen Excess Society (AES) advocated that all of the signs and symptoms should be present for the confirmation of diagnose [6] (**Table 1**).

Contrary to physicians' and patients' belief, weight or body mass index (BMI) had never been a part of PCOs definition.

NIH Criteria 1990 (all of them)	ESHRE[1]/ASRM[2] (Rotterdam) 2003 (two of three)	AES 2006 (all of them)
Hyperandrogenism ± hyperandrogenemia	Hyperandrogenism±hyperandrogenemia	Hyperandrogenism ± hyperandrogenemia
Oligo-ovulation	Menstruation abnormality	Ovarian dysfunction ± sonographic aspect
	Sonographic aspect of poly cystic ovary	

Exclusion of other androgen excess conditions is necessary for all of definition: (21-hydroxylase deficient, thyroid dysfunction, nonclassical adrenal hyperplasia, hyper prolactinemia, drug-induced androgen excess, androgenic neoplasm, Cushing syndrome, growth hormone excess).
[1]European Society for Human Reproductive Medicine.
[2]American Society for Reproductive Medicine.

Table 1. Different definition of polycystic ovary syndrome.

According to epidemiological data, there is a wide variation in the prevalence of obese and non-obese PCOs women: in Korean population 20%, in Europe 27–50.5%, and in USA 67% of PCOs woman are obese [7–11]. Regarding to different ethnicity, the prevalence of normal weight and underweight patients with PCOs has been reported 1.5–6.6% [12, 13]. Entirely, by using Rotterdam criteria, the overall prevalence of PCOs is increasing because ovulatory or non-hyper androgen PCO patients also are considered [14].

By definition, women with BMI ≤ 25 are non-obese and with BMI > 25 considered obese.

Although at now, we have a few reports about the prevalence of non-obese PCOs patients, but attention toward those patients and their metabolic and health problems are enhanced day by day.

The pathophysiology of PCOs is multifactorial and manifests the final effect of genetic, fetal, environmental, and metabolic factors. As a result of weakness or strength of each factor, clinical and subclinical character and their response to therapeutic efforts will be different.

2. Genetic and PCOs

Obvious familial clustering of PCOs and higher prevalence of its sign and symptom, like type 2 diabetes mellitus (T2DM) and hyperandrogenemia in first-degree relatives of women with PCOs, demonstrate its genetic origin [15, 16]. Also, in the Dutch twin study, higher degree of heritability was shown [17]. Initially, autosomal dominant mode of inheritance was suggested [18]; but after a while, researches demonstrate it has more complex inheritance pattern. Despite the progress in genes or loci study, no single gene has been successfully described as the certain responsible gene among all studies [19]. According to microarray analysis results, 14 important genes were recognized: 6 genes were identified as down-regulated genes and 8 genes as up-regulated genes [20]. Another proposed genes are *CYP11A*, the insulin gene, and a region near the insulin-receptor gene [21]. Also, controlling genes in folliculogenesis and LH receptor and coding genes for TNF-alpha, IL-6, and IL-6 receptor can be involved in the pathogenesis of this syndrome [22].

3. Insulin and PCOs

For the first time in 1980, the relation between this syndrome and insulin was determinate [23]. Clinically insulin resistance (IR) is specified as inability of a known amount of endogenous or exogenous insulin to enhance glucose uptake and consumption. As a result of a misbelief that IR always accompanies with obesity, in clinical practice, IR is underestimated in non-obese PCO women. IR is a common character between obese and non-obese PCO patients and its overall prevalence is 50–75%. Up to 35% of PCOs women have IGTT and 7–10% are type 2 diabetes mellitus (T2DM) [24].

At now, the most used IR indices are homeostasis-model assessment (HOMA) and insulinemic 2-h area under the curve (AUCi 2 h), both derived from oral glucose tolerance test (OGTT) [25]. The 120-min glucose and insulin evaluation (HOMA-M_{120}) is the best IR index in lean PCOs women according to Morciano et al. study [26]. Meanwhile, there are several earlier studies about IR evaluation in lean PCOs women [27–29]. Although, a study in a large group of European lean PCOs patients displayed that this group had significantly less IR compared with obese PCO women [30]; but, instead of it, there is evidence that in American and Asian PCOs women, IR is independent from BMI [31]. It seems that dietary composition and ethnic background associated with this discrepancy.

Owing to another recent study, the crucial role of insulin in PCO pathogenesis emphasized that IR shall be evaluated even in normal weight and lean PCOs patients [12].

As suggested in the earlier study [32], hyperinsulinemia stimulates ovarian P450c17 alpha activity in non-obese women with PCOs, which means more conversion of progesterone to androstenedione which is changed to testosterone. In granulosa cell, insulin intensifies their response to LH. Therefore, these cells experience premature arrest of follicular growth and abnormal differentiation, and thus anovulation. Also, elevated insulin resistance causes hyperglycemia which leads to hyperinsulinemia and it can increase LH action on theca cells and subsequent elevation in androgen level. Hyperinsulinemia, insulin resistance, and enhancement in androgen production are the famous pathophysiology triads in PCOs. From another side, elevated level of insulin prevents hepatic sex hormone-binding globulin (SHBG) production, which can lead to elevated free androgen and again elevated level of insulin, a positive feedback in an undesirable circle. Thus, IR and hyperinsulinemia are the principal pathological causes of this syndrome, and hyperandrogenemia is their consequence.

As insulin resistance has fundamental role in non-obese PCOs patients, then metformin administration have a beneficial effect on them and regulate their menstruation cycle [33]. As well, there is a new therapeutic option: inositol, a precursor component of second messenger for follicle-stimulating hormone (FSH), *thyroid - stimulating hormone* (TSH), and insulin receptor. This drug can overcome IR from another way [34]. It is important to mention that only 15% of women with IR are having PCOs criteria; therefore, insulin resistance cannot be the only pathophysiologic pathway [35] and metformin administration may not be effective in all of lean PCOs.

4. Androgens and PCO

About 10–12% of women in reproductive age suffer from androgen excess sign and symptom. It can be caused by androgen overproduction (from ovary or adrenal gland) or secondary to increased sensitivity of pilosebaceous unit (with normal level of androgens). Hyperandrogenemia is another hallmark of PCOs; mainly by ovarian resource and less by adrenal. In PCOs women, 60% of serum androstenedione and testosterone (T) are secreted by ovary. Surprising, ovarian androgens will not prominently affect LH production, thus an elevation in free testosterone or androstenedione will not decrease ovarian synthesis of these androgens in women, contrasting to men.

As mentioned before, in PCO women, insulin in a solitary manner or with synergetic effect of LH induces androgen production by ovaries. Even in lean PCOs women with normal metabolic insulin sensitivity and insulin levels, decline of insulin secretion with diazoxide (like metformin) prominently reduce levels of free T and androstenedione and meaningfully increased SHBG [36]. In these women, hyperandrogenemia is seen because of augmented sensitivity of their androgenic pathway to insulin and dysregulation of steroidogeneses enzymes based on genetic predisposition [37]. Therefore, even in PCOs patients with normal insulin metabolic and without clinical approved IR, local resistance in the ovaries increased androgens production [38].

Androgen excess or hyperandrogenemia (HA) in PCOs women contribute in exacerbation of metabolic abnormalities, such as insulin resistance in adipose tissue and skeletal muscle and elevation in lipid metabolism in visceral fat, decreased lipolysis in subcutaneous fat, increased low-density lipoprotein cholesterol (LDL-C) levels decreased HDL-C levels. Besides that, androgens may be involved in possible direct vascular action [39]. There are some studies, in which hyperandrogenemia was accompanying with metabolic syndrome (MetS) in non-obese PCOs more than obese PCOs women [40, 41].

Hyperandrogenemia or androgen access clinical signs are mainly cutaneous manifestations: hirsutism, acne, androgenic alopecia, acanthosis nigricans (AN), and seborrhea. In one study, their prevalence in PCOs women was: 78, 48, 31, 30, and 29% (in mentioned order) [42]. In another study, the prevalence of acanthosis nigricans in obese PCO was 42.5% compared to 28% in non-obese [43]. One published paper shows that AN is a marker of hyperinsulinemia in both obese and non-obese PCO patients rather than a sign of androgen excess and the only sex steroid associated with histological AN is dehydroepiandrosterone sulfate (DHEAS) [44].

Pharmacological management of hyperandrogenic skin symptoms has two targets: firstly, decrease the level of circulating androgens, and secondly prevent their effect at tissue level. Cyproterone acetate/ethinylestradiol has beneficial effect in non-obese PCO women with hyperandrogenic skin symptoms [45].

5. Inflammation and PCO

There are many published studies about proinflammatory or inflammatory situations in PCOs woman. Increased level of circulatory inflammatory markers like C-reactive protein (CRP), tumor necrosis factor-alpha (TNF-α), interleukins (IL-16 and -18), and plasminogen activator inhibitor in PCO patients accompany with abdominal obesity and more specific with visceral fat [46]. Low-grade inflammation situation by increased level of adiponectin, resistin, IL-6, and TNF-α in non-obese PCO women have been approved [47]. Also, it has been shown that inhibition of nutrient-induced inflammation decreases ovarian androgen secretion and induces ovulation in lean PCOs woman without clinical IR or abdominal adiposity. Therefore, inflammation directly encourages ovarian dysfunction in PCOs women distinctly from insulin resistance or excess adiposity [48]. There is evidence that non-steroidal anti-inflammatory agent administration in lean PCO women can reduce androgen secretion from ovary [49].

Dose inflammation have pathophysiologic role in this syndrome or may be its consequence remain still unclear. Inflammation as a chronic immune activation, prevents ovulation, increases androgen production by ovary and adrenal gland and disrupts hormonal receptors. Most of long-term complications of PCOs like cardiovascular disease (CVD) are consequences of inflammatory state [50].

In non-obese PCO patients, visceral fat distribution, waist to hip ratio (WHR), and abdominal obesity have relation with inflammatory situation. In one study, in lean PCOs, level of white blood cell (WBC) has a positive predictive value with insulin resistance, while the neutrophil to lymphocyte ratio has a negative predictive value [51]. Also, it has been demonstrated that in clomiphene citrate (CC)-resistant patients, regardless to BMI, inflammatory markers like TNF-α are too high, and TNF-α serum level may be used as a clinical predictive indicator before CC useless administration [52].

6. Weight and PCO

Even in lean PCO women, we can see higher waist to hip ratio, greater intra peritoneal and visceral fat, and percentage of body fat in comparison with BMI matched non-PCO women. Accumulation of small subcutaneous abdominal fat in those patients shows spoiled adipogenesis and hyperandrogenism [53]. Also, abnormal gene expression in stem cell of subcutaneous abdominal fat in normoandrogen and ovulatory lean PCO women display abnormal vacuolization and angiogenesis, which may reflect metabolism alter in those women [54]. From another side, adiponectin, a protein which is involved in regulating glucose levels and fatty acid breakdown, is produced by omental fat and dysregulated by high level of insulin; thus, even in lean PCOs women, inappropriate metabolism of glucose and lipid can be explained [55]. In respect with a new randomized controlled trial, arranged and regular physical exercise can ameliorate insulin sensitivity, hyperandrogenemia, and menstrual regularity in lean PCO women [56].

7. Metabolic disorders and PCO

PCOs is considered by multiple metabolic disorders which may associate to increase risk of hypertension and cardiovascular disease. One study used menstrual irregularity as a predictive factor for assessment of cardiovascular events in a 15-year period, in PCOs women. There was an insignificant increase in overall stroke risk and in ischemic stroke risk associated with "very irregular" menstrual cycles [57]. In PCO women, higher prevalence of hypertension is related to insulin. Hyperinsulinemia have been connected with an increase in intracellular sodium and calcium, along with vascular smooth muscle hypertrophy due to insulin-like growth factor-1 (IGF-1) activity [58]. Simultaneously, androgen excess stimulates sympathetic nerve activity, as another etiology of hypertension in this population [59].

PCOs is also associated with elevated levels of plasma endothelin-1 (ET-1), one of several circulating indicators of endothelial injury and dysfunction. One study found that impairment of endothelial function is more severe in lean than obese women with PCOs, and that ET receptor downregulation plays an essential role in this probably adverse cardiovascular outcome [60].

The increase in carotid intima-media wall thickness (CIMT) in PCOs women has been associated in different studies with higher levels of insulin, hyperandrogenism, LDL level, and abdominal obesity; which is an early marker of atherosclerosis [61].

Meanwhile, impaired nitric oxide (NO) production as a consequence of elevated androgen levels in PCOs women contribute to endothelial dysfunction [62].

Elevated plasma viscosity as a result of increased plasma fibrinogen concentration in PCOs patients exacerbates vascular dysfunction because autoregulation of vasomotor tone may not be able to adjust with compromised physical properties of blood [63]. Some possible reasons for increased plasma fibrinogen are: increased inflammatory processes [64], decreased fibrinolysis [65], and as an acute phase reactant. Enhancement in fibrinogen level stimulates RBC aggregation and significantly increased resistance in blood flow [66]. Low SHBG and high insulin stimulate prothrombotic state in all of PCOs women by increased plasminogen activator inhibitor 1 (PAI-1) activity and fibrinogen in a BMI-independent way [67].

Dyslipidemia including elevated low-density lipoprotein (LDL), triglyceride levels and decreased high-density lipoprotein (HDL) are often seen in PCO women as a result of hyperandrogenism and insulin resistance in both lean and obese PCO patients [68].

Owing to many evidence about vitamin D deficiency and metabolic syndrome; there are many studies about 25(OH) D levels and PCOs. There are some evidences which support this relationship and encourage vitamin D administration in all of deficient PCOs women [69], whereas some studies do not support it [70].

From another site, insulin resistance, increased central adiposity, higher levels of testosterone, and dyslipidemia beside oxidative stress and low grade inflammation contribute to cause hepatic steatosis or fatty liver in PCOs women. Advanced stage of this disease characterized by necrosis and steatohepatitis which called non-alcoholic fatty liver disease (NAFLD) and has prevalence about 40% in lean PCOs women [71].

After blow-by-blow discussion about all of aspects in lean PCOs women, we cannot consider this syndrome as just a part of infertility or menstrual abnormality assessment, but should be accepted as an alarm sign for serious health problem.

Author details

Elham Pourmatroud

Address all correspondence to: e.pourmatroud@yahoo.com

Sarem Women Hospital, Tehran, Iran

References

[1] Azziz R, Woods KS, Reyna R, Key TJ, Knochenhauer ES, Yildiz BO. The prevalence and features of the polycystic ovary syndrome in an unselected population. The Journal of Clinical Endocrinology and Metabolism. 2004;**89**(6):2745-2749. DOI: 10.1210/jc.2003-032046

[2] Botsis D, Kassanos D, Pyrgiotis E, Zourlas PA. Sonographic incidence of polycystic ovaries in a gynecological population. Ultrasound in Obstetrics & Gynecology. 1995;**6**(3): 182-185. DOI: 10.1046/j.1469-0705.1995.06030182.x

[3] Stein IF, Leventhal ML. Amenorrhea associated with bilateral polycystic ovaries. American Journal of Obstetrics and Gynecology. 1935;**29**(2):181-191. DOI: http://dx.doi.org/10.1016/S0002-9378(15)30642-6

[4] Roe AH, Dokras A. The diagnosis of polycystic ovary syndrome in adolescents. Reviews in Obstetrics & Gynecology. 2011;**4**(2):45-51 PMCID: PMC3218544

[5] The Rotterdam ESHRE/ASRM-sponsored PCOS Consensus Workshop Group 2004 Revised 2003 consensus on diagnostic criteria and long-term health risks related to polycystic ovary syndrome (PCOS). Human Reproduction. 2004;**19**(1):41-47 PMID: 14688154

[6] Azziz R, Carmina E, Dewailly D, Diamanti-Kandarakis E, Escobar-Morreale HF, Futterweit W, et al. The Androgen Excess and PCOS Society criteria for the polycystic ovary syndrome: the complete task force report. Fertility and Sterility. 2009;**91**(2):456-488. DOI: 10.1016/j.fertnstert.2008.06.035

[7] Carmina E, Legro RS, Stamets K, Lowell J, Lobo RA. Difference in body weight between American and Italian women with polycystic ovary syndrome: Influence of the diet. Human Reproduction. 2003;**18**(11):2289-2293 PMID: 14585875

[8] Diamanti-Kandarakis E, Kouli CR, Bergiele AT, Filandra FA, Tsianateli TC, Spina GG, et al. A survey of the polycystic ovary syndrome in the Greek island of Lesbos: Hormonal and metabolic profile. The Journal of Clinical Endocrinology and Metabolism. 1999;**84**(11): 4006-4011. DOI: doi.org/10.1210/jcem.84.11.6148

[9] Knochenhauer ES, Key TJ, Kahsar-Miller M, Waggoner W, Boots LR, Azziz R. Prevalence of the polycystic ovary syndrome in unselected black and white women of the southeastern United States: A prospective study. The Journal of Clinical Endocrinology and Metabolism. 1998;**83**(9):3078-3082. DOI: 10.1210/jcem.83.9.5090

[10] Kim JJ, Hwang KR, Choi YM, Moon SY, Chae SJ, Park CW, et al. Complete phenotypic and metabolic profiles of a large consecutive cohort of untreated Korean women with polycystic ovary syndrome. Fertility and Sterility. 2014;**101**(5):1424-1430. DOI: 10.1016/j.fertnstert.2014.01.049

[11] Kyrkou G, Trakakis E, Attilakos A, Panagopoulos P, Chrelias C, Papadimitriou A, et al. Metabolic syndrome in Greek women with polycystic ovary syndrome: Prevalence, characteristics and associations with body mass index. A prospective controlled study. Archives of Gynecology and Obstetrics. 2016;**293**(4):915-923. DOI: 10.1007/s00404-015-3964-y

[12] Anastasiou OE, Canbay A, Fuhrer D, Reger-Tan S. Metabolic and androgen profile in underweight women with polycystic ovary syndrome. Archives of Gynecology and Obstetrics. 2017;**296**(2):363-371. DOI: 10.1007/s00404-017-4422-9

[13] Sheng Y, Lu G, Liu J, Liang X, Ma Y, Zhang X, et al. Effect of body mass index on the outcomes of controlled ovarian hyperstimulation in Chinese women with polycystic ovary syndrome: A multicenter, prospective, observational study. Journal of Assisted Reproduction and Genetics. 2017;**34**(1):61-70. DOI: 10.1007/s10815-016-0830-1

[14] March WA, Moore VM, Willson KJ, Phillips DI, Norman RJ, Davies MJ. The prevalence of polycystic ovary syndrome in a community sample assessed under contrasting diagnostic criteria. Human Reproduction. 2010;**25**(2):544-551. DOI: 10.1093/humrep/dep399

[15] Ehrmann DA, Kasza K, Azziz R, Legro RS, Ghazzi MN. Effects of race and family history of type 2 diabetes on metabolic status of women with polycystic ovary syndrome. The Journal of Clinical Endocrinology and Metabolism. 2005;**90**:66-71. DOI: 10.1210/jc.2004-0229

[16] Legro RS, Driscoll D, Strauss JF 3rd, Fox J, Dunaif A. Evidence for a genetic basis for hyperandrogenemia in polycystic ovary syndrome. Proceedings of the National Academy of Sciences of the United States of America. 1998;**95**:14956-14960 PMCID: PMC24557

[17] Vink JM, Sadrzadeh S, Lambalk CB, Boomsma DI. Heritability of polycystic ovary syndrome in a Dutch twin-family study. The Journal of Clinical Endocrinology and Metabolism. 2006;**91**:2100-2104. DOI: 10.1210/jc.2005-1494

[18] Govind A, Obhrai MS, Clayton RN. Polycystic ovaries are inherited as an autosomal dominant trait: Analysis of 29 polycystic ovary syndrome and 10 control families. The Journal of Clinical Endocrinology and Metabolism. 1999;**84**(1):38-43. DOI: 10.1210/jcem.84.1.5382

[19] Kosova G, Urbanek M. Genetics of the polycystic ovary syndrome. Molecular and Cellular Endocrinology. 2013;**373**:29-38. DOI: 10.1016/j.mce.2012.10.009

[20] Panda PK, Rane R, Ravichandran R, Singh S, Panchal H. Genetics of PCOS: A systematic bioinformatics approach to unveil the proteins responsible for PCOS. Genomics Data. 2016;**8**:52-60. DOI: 10.1016/j.gdata.2016.03.008

[21] Legro RS, Strauss JF. Molecular progress in infertility: Polycystic ovary syndrome. Fertility and Sterility. 2002;**78**:569-576 PMID: 12215335

[22] De Leo V, Musacchio MC, Cappelli V, Massaro MG, Morgante G, Petraglia F. Genetic, hormonal and metabolic aspects of PCOS: An update. Reproductive Biology and Endocrinology. 2016;**14**(1):38-50. DOI: 10.1186/s12958-016-0173-x

[23] Burghen GA, Givens JR, Kitabchi AE. Correlation of hyperandrogenism with hyperinsulinism in polycystic ovarian disease. The Journal of Clinical Endocrinology and Metabolism. 1980;**50**:113-116. DOI: 10.1210/jcem-50-1-113

[24] O'Meara NM, Blackman JD, Ehrmann DA, Barnes RB, Jaspan JB, Rosenfield RL, Polonsky KS. Defects in beta-cell function in functional ovarian hyperandrogenism. The Journal of Clinical Endocrinology and Metabolism. 1993;**76**(5):1241-1247. DOI: 10.1210/jcem.76.5.8496316

[25] Bonora E, Targher G, Alberiche M, Bonadonna RC, Saggiani F, Zenere MB, et al. Homeostasis model assessment closely mirrors the glucose clamp technique in the assessment of insulin sensitivity: Studies in subjects with various degrees of glucose tolerance and insulin sensitivity. Diabetes Care. 2000;**23**:57-63 PMID: 10857969

[26] Morciano A, Romani F, Sagnella F, Scarinci E, Palla C, Moro F, et al. Assessment of insulin resistance in lean women with polycystic ovary syndrome. Fertility and Sterility. 2014;**102**(1): 250-256. DOI: 10.1016/j.fertnstert.2014.04.004

[27] Dunaif A, Segal KR, Shelley DR, Green G, Dobrjansky A, Licholai T. Evidence for distinctive and intrinsic defects in insulin action in polycystic ovary syndrome. Diabetes. 1992;**41**:1257-1266 PMID: 1397698

[28] Chang RJ, Nakamura RM, Judd HL, Kaplan SA. Insulin resistance in nonobese patients with polycystic ovarian disease. The Journal of Clinical Endocrinology and Metabolism. 1983;**57**:356-359. DOI: 10.1210/jcem-57-2-356

[29] Dunaif A, Segal KR, Futterweit W, Dobrjansky A. Profound peripheral insulin resistance, independent of obesity, in polycystic ovary syndrome. Diabetes. 1989;**38**:1165-1174 PMID: 2670645

[30] Vrbikova J, Cibula D, Dvorakova K, Stanicka S, Sindelka G, Hill M, et al. Insulin sensitivity in women with polycystic ovary syndrome. The Journal of Clinical Endocrinology and Metabolism. 2004;**89**:2942-2945. DOI: 10.1210/jc.2003-031378

[31] Takeuchi T, Tsutsumi O, Taketani Y. Abnormal response of insulin to glucose loading and assessment of insulin resistance in nonobese patients with polycystic ovary syndrome. Gynecological Endocrinology. 2008;**24**:385-391. DOI: 10.1080/09513590802173584

[32] Nestler JE, Jakubowicz DJ. Lean women with polycystic ovary syndrome respond to insulin reduction with decreases in ovarian P450c17 alpha activity and serum androgens. The Journal of Clinical Endocrinology and Metabolism. 1997;**82**(12):4075-4079. DOI: 10.1210/jcem.82.12.4431

[33] Al-Ozairi E, Quinton R, Advani A. Therapeutic response to metformin in an underweight patient with polycystic ovarian syndrome. Fertility and Sterility. 2008;**90**(4):1197.e1-1197.e4. DOI: 10.1016/j.fertnstert.2007.11.041

[34] Genazzani AD. Inositol as putative integrative treatment for PCOS. Reproductive Biomedicine Online. 2016;**33**(6):770-780. DOI: 10.1016/j.rbmo.2016.08.024

[35] Barbieri RL, Smith S, Ryan KJ. The role of hyperinsulinemia in the pathogenesis of ovarian hyperandrogenism. Fertility and Sterility. 1988;**50**(2):197-212 PMID: 3294042

[36] Baillargeon JP, Carpentier A. Role of insulin in the hyperandrogenemia of lean women with polycystic ovary syndrome and normal insulin sensitivity. Fertility and Sterility. 2007;**88**(4):10-16. DOI: 10.1016/j.fertnstert.2006.12.055

[37] Jakimiuk AJ, Weitsman SR, Navab A, Magoffin DA. Luteinizing hormone receptor, steroidogenesis acute regulatory protein, and steroidogenic enzyme messenger ribonucleic acids are overexpressed in thecal and granulosa cells from polycystic ovaries. The Journal of Clinical Endocrinology and Metabolism. 2001;**86**(3):1318-1323. DOI: 10.1210/jcem.86.3.7318

[38] Wu XK, Zhou SY, Liu JX, Pollanen P, Sallinen K, Makinen M, et al. Selective ovary resistance to insulin signaling in women with polycystic ovary syndrome. Fertility and Sterility. 2003;**80**:954-965 PMID: 14556818

[39] Christakou CD, Diamanti-Kandarakis E. Role of androgen excess on metabolic aberrations and cardiovascular risk in women with polycystic ovary syndrome. Women's Health. 2009;**4**:583-594. DOI: 10.2217/17455057.4.6.583

[40] Mehrabian F, Khani B, Kelishadi R, Kermani N. The prevalence of metabolic syndrome and insulin resistance according to the phenotypic subgroups of polycystic ovary syndrome in a representative sample of Iranian females. Journal of Research in Medical Sciences. 2011;**16**:763-769 PMCID: PMC3214394

[41] Kim MJ, Lim NK, Choi YM, Kim JJ, Hwang KR, Chae SJ, et al. Prevalence of metabolic syndrome is higher among non-obese PCOS women with hyperandrogenism and menstrual irregularity in Korea. PloS One. 2014;**9**(6):e99252. DOI: 10.1371/journal.pone.0099252

[42] Abid Keen M, Hassan Shah I, Sheikh G. Cutaneous manifestations of polycystic ovary syndrome: A cross-sectional clinical study. Indian Dermatology Online Journal. 2017;**8**(2):104-110. DOI: 10.4103/2229-5178.202275

[43] IbrahimMahmoud M, Habeebc F, Kasim K. Reproductive and biochemical changes in obese and non-obese polycystic ovary syndrome women. Alexandria Journal of Medicine. 2015;**51**(1):5-9. DOI: doi.org/10.1016/j.ajme.2014.03.002

[44] Dunaif A, Green G, Phelps RG, Lebwohl M, Futterweit W, Lewy L. Acanthosis Nigricans, insulin action, and hyperandrogenism: Clinical, histological, and biochemical findings. The Journal of Clinical Endocrinology and Metabolism. 1991;**73**(3):590-595. DOI: 10.1210/jcem-73-3-590

[45] Bitzer J, Römer T, Lopes da Silva Filho A. The use of Cyproterone acetate/ethinyl estradiol in hyperandrogenic skin symptoms—A review. The European Journal of Contraception & Reproductive Health Care. 2017;**22**(3):172-182. DOI: dx.doi.org/10.1080/13625187.2017.1317339

[46] Bruun JM, Lihn AS, Pedersen SB, Richelsen B. Monocyte chemoattractant protein-1 release is higher in visceral than subcutaneous human adipose tissue (AT): Implication of macrophages resident in the AT. The Journal of Clinical Endocrinology and Metabolism. 2005;**90**(4):2282-2289. DOI: 10.1210/jc.2004-1696

[47] Y-X WANG, W-J ZHU. Evaluation of adiponectin, resistin, IL-6, TNF-α in obese and non-obese women with polycystic ovary syndrome. Journal of Reproduction and Contraception. 2012;**23**(4):237-244. DOI: doi.org/10.1016/S1001-7844(12)60032-7

[48] Gonzalez F, Mather KJ, Considine RV, Pardue SL, Acton AJ. Suppression of nutrient-induced inflammation with a nonsteroidal anti-inflammatory agent ameliorates ovarian dysfunction in lean insulin-sensitive women with polycystic ovary syndrome (PCOS). Fertility and Sterility. 2015;**14**(3):e21. DOI: 10.1016/j.fertnstert.2015.07.064

[49] Gonzalez F, Considine RV, Abdelhadi OA, Acton AJ. Anti-inflammatory therapy suppresses proinflammatory cytokine secretion from mononuclear cells and reduces hyperandrogenism in lean women with polycystic ovary syndrome (PCOS). Fertility and Sterility. 2016;**106**(3):e32. DOI: 10.1016/j.fertnstert.2016.07.104

[50] Hyderali BN, Mala K. Oxidative stress and cardiovascular complications in polycystic ovarian syndrome. European Journal of Obstetrics, Gynecology, and Reproductive Biology. 2015;**191**:15-22. DOI: 10.1016/j.ejogrb.2015.05.005

[51] Tola EN, Yalcin SE, Dugan N. The predictive effect of inflammatory markers and lipid accumulation product index on clinical symptoms associated with polycystic ovary syndrome in non-obese adolescents and younger aged women. European Journal of Obstetrics, Gynecology, and Reproductive Biology. 2017;**214**:168-172. DOI: 10.1016/j.ejogrb.2017.05.014

[52] Seyam E, Hasan M, Khalifa EM, Ramadn A, Hefzy E. Evaluation of tumor necrosis factor alpha serum level in obese and lean women with clomiphene citrate-resistant polycystic ovary disease. Gynecological Endocrinology. 2017;**8**:1-7. DOI: 10.1080/09513590.2017.1320383

[53] Akopians AL, Madrigal V, Fisch S, Ramirez E, Margolis D, Sarma MK, et al. Hyperandro genism is associated with preferential fat deposition of visceral versus subcutaneous (SC) abdominal fat in lean polycystic ovary syndrome (PCOS) women. Fertility and Sterility. 2016;**106**(3):Supp:e31-Supp:e32. DOI: 10.1016/j.fertnstert.2016.07.102

[54] Phan J, Madrigal VK, Guedikian A, Li X, Dumesic DA, Chazenbalk GD. Immunological, structural and stem cell characteristics of subcutaneous (SC) abdominal adipose in lean polycystic ovary syndrome (PCOS) women versus normoandrogenic ovulatory (NL) women. Fertility and Sterility. 2016;**106**(3):supp:e250. DOI: 10.1016/j.fertnstert.2016.07.722

[55] Seow KM, Tsai YL, Juan CC, Lin YH, Hwang JL, Ho LT. Omental fat expression of adiponectin and adiponectin receptors in non-obese women with PCOS: A preliminary study. Reproductive Biomedicine Online. 2009;**19**(4):577-582 PMID:19909601

[56] Bisgaard H, Dela F. Physical exercise is a help for lean women with polycystic ovary syndrome. Ugeskrift for Laeger. 2017;**179**(23): PMID: 28606299

[57] Solomon CG, Hu FB, Dunaif A, Rich-Edwards JE, Stampfer MJ, Willett WC, et al. Menstrual cycle irregularity and risk for future cardiovascular disease. The J Clin Endocrinol Metab. 2002 May;**87**(5):2013-17. DOI: 10.1210/jcem.87.5.8471

[58] Zavaroni I, Coruzzi P, Bonini L, Mossini GL, Musiari L, Gasparini P, et al. Association between salt sensitivity and insulin concentrations in patients with hypertension. American Journal of Hypertension. 1995;**8**(8):855-858. DOI: 10.1016/0895-7061(95)00152-F

[59] Sverrisdottir YB, Mogren T, Kataoka J, Janson PO, Stener-Victorin E. Is polycystic ovary syndrome associated with high sympathetic nerve activity and size at birth? American Journal of Physiology. Endocrinology and Metabolism. 2008;**294**:E576-E581. DOI: 10.1152/ajpendo.00725.2007

[60] Usselman CW, Taylor HS, Stachenfeld NS. Microvascular endothelial function in lean versus obese women with polycystic ovary syndrome: Role of the endothelin B receptor. Gynecological Endocrinology. 2007;**23**(10):604-609. DOI: 10.1096/fj.1530-6860

[61] Baldani DP, Skrgatic L, Ougouag R. Polycystic ovary syndrome: Important underrecognised cardiometabolic risk factor in reproductive-age women. International Journal of Endocrinology. 2015;**786362**. DOI: 10.1155/2015/786362

[62] Paradisi G, Steinberg HO, Hempfling A, et al. Polycystic ovary syndrome is associated with endothelial dysfunction. Circulation. 2001;**103**(10):1410-1415 PMID: 11245645

[63] Vervita V, Saltamavros AD, Adonakis G, Tsapanos V, Decavalas G, Georgopoulos NA. Obesity and insulin resistance increase plasma viscosity in young women with polycystic ovary syndrome. Gynecological Endocrinology: The Official Journal of the International Society of Gynecological Endocrinology. 2009;**25**(10):640-646. DOI: 10.1371/journal.pone.0167290

[64] Gonzalez F. Inflammation in polycystic ovary syndrome: Underpinning of insulin resistance and ovarian dysfunction. Steroids. 2012;**77**(4):300-305. DOI: 10.1016/j.steroids.2011.12.003

[65] Burchall GF, Piva TJ, Linden MD, Gibson-Helm ME, Ranasinha S, Teede HJ. Comprehensive assessment of the hemostatic system in polycystic ovarian syndrome. Seminars in Thrombosis and Hemostasis. 2015. DOI: 10.1055/s-0035-1564837

[66] Simmonds MJ, Milne N, Ong K, Brotherton E, McNamee AP, Horobin J, Sabapathy S. Physical properties of blood are altered in young and lean women with polycystic ovary syndrome. PLoS One. 2016;**11**(11):e0167290. DOI: 10.1371/journal.pone.0167290

[67] Manneràs-Holm L, Baghaei F, Holm G, Janson PO, Ohlsson C, Lönn M, Stener-Victorin E. Coagulation and fibrinolytic disturbances in women with polycystic ovary syndrome.

The Journal of Clinical Endocrinology and Metabolism. 2011;**96**(4):1068-1076. DOI: 10.1210/jc.2010-2279

[68] Yildirim B, Sabir N, Kaleli B. Relation of intra-abdominal fat distribution to metabolic disorders in nonobese patients with polycystic ovary syndrome. Fertility and Sterility. 2003;**79**(6):1358-1364 PMID:12798883

[69] Wehr E, Pilz S, Schweighofer N, Giuliani A, Kopera D, Pieber TR, Obermayer-Pietsch B. Association of hypovitaminosis D with metabolic disturbances in polycystic ovary syndrome. European Journal of Endocrinology. 2009;**161**(4):575-582. DOI: 10.1530/EJE-09-0432

[70] Rashidi H, Najafian M, Toolabi M, Safapoor N, Sadrian E, Nazari P. The relationship of serum 25-dihydroxy vitamin D3 concentrations with metabolic parameters in non-obese women with polycystic ovarian syndrome. Middle East Fertility Society Journal. 2016; **21**(4):264-268. DOI: 10.1016/j.mefs.2016.06.003

[71] Gambarin-Gelwan M, Kinkhabwala SV, Schiano TD, Bodian C, Yeh HC, Futterweit W. Prevalence of nonalcoholic fatty liver disease in women with polycystic ovary syndrome. Clinical Gastroenterology and Hepatology. 2007;**5**(4):496-501. DOI: 10.1016/j.cgh.2006.10.010

Section 3

Therapy for Polycystic Ovarian Disease

Chapter 4

Lifestyle Changes and Weight Loss: Effects in PCOS

Cringu Antoniu Ionescu, Ina Popescu,
Mihail Banacu and Mihai Dimitriu

Additional information is available at the end of the chapter

http://dx.doi.org/10.5772/intechopen.73298

Abstract

Even though controversies surrounding the polycystic ovary syndrome are not yet close to be solved, its clinical manifestations are well known—insulin resistance and obesity, hirsutism, irregular and anovulatory menstrual cycles. The treatment of polycystic ovarian syndrome (PCOS) is mainly symptomatic as its etiology is not yet clear. Lifestyle changes are the primary therapy in overweight and obese women with PCOS. According to majority of the studies, lifestyle changes are the most effective form of treatment not only for weight loss but also for the improvement of insulin sensitivity, decreasing incidence of metabolic syndrome and type 2 diabetes. Studies also show that weight loss has fertility benefits by restoring ovulatory cycles. Although initial studies researching pharmacologic treatment were showing excellent results concerning the weight loss, maintenance of weight loss and reduction of cardiovascular risks, some of these drugs were in the end, has proven to actually increase the risk for cardiovascular events and were removed from the market. Bariatric surgery has been demonstrated to improve or even cure type 2 diabetes, hypertension, hyperlipidemia, and obstructive sleep apnea. More so, there are studies that reported complete resolution of all features of PCOS, even hirsutism, hyperandrogenism, anovulation, and menstrual irregularity.

Keywords: polycystic ovarian syndrome (PCOS), obesity, hyperandrogenism, anovulation, hirsutism, metabolic syndrome, weight loss

1. Introduction

Polycystic ovary syndrome (PCOS) is considered to be the most common endocrinopathy affecting women with an incidence ranging from 5 to 13% [1], depending on the diagnostic criteria applied.

Polycystic ovary syndrome—in spite of many years of research—is still a controversial topic. We have come to know in detail its clinical manifestations such as metabolic disorders, menstrual and ovulatory dysfunctions, and clinical hyperandrogenism. However, not knowing its etiology, most of the treatments suggested to patients with PCOS are symptomatic, not addressing to the underlying cause, but rather each symptom in part.

Following numerous studies and research on PCOS and despite that the exact mechanism is not completely understood, the conclusions of most researchers are the same; lifestyle change and weight loss have beneficial effects on the entire panel of symptoms associated with this syndrome.

2. Which are the main goals when treating PCOS?

2.1. Management of underlying metabolic disorders, reduction of risk factors for type 2 diabetes and cardiovascular disease

2.1.1. Obesity

Under the metabolic disorders, which are commonly encountered in patients with PCOS, it is worth mentioning: obesity, insulin resistance, metabolic syndrome, dyslipidemia, and type 2 diabetes mellitus.

Some researchers state that the obesity rate in the case of the women with PCOS is even up to 70%, but most agree that at least half of the women with PCOS suffer from obesity (body mass index (BMI) = 19–25 kg/m^2) [2] and in most cases, it is of a central distribution (waist circumference > 88 cm) [3]. Of the nonobese patients, one-third has increased intra-abdominal fat [4]. There is no specific data on why the prevalence of obesity is much higher in women with PCOS, but most researchers attribute it to the hyperinsulinemia resulting from the insulin resistance, an important factor of adipogenesis, lipogenesis, and lipolysis inhibition [5].

2.1.2. Increased insulin resistance

Insulin resistance and reactive hyperinsulinemia are definitely implicated in the physiopathological mechanism of PCOS. With respect to insulin resistance, some authors consider it to be uncorrelated to the degree of the obesity [6], while others argue that the obesity, especially the central one, seems to increase the metabolic and clinical features of insulin resistance [7]. Although obese patients seem to be more affected by insulin resistance, this also occurs in the cases of nonobese patients with PCOS [8].

2.1.3. Metabolic syndrome

The metabolic syndrome is commonly associated with PCOS, with a prevalence ranging between 33 and 47% [9]. Both PCOS and the metabolic syndrome have features that generate an increased risk of cardiovascular diseases–if this risk is independent of PCOS or it is caused by its association with the metabolic syndrome, it is still a topic of debate [10]. Studies demonstrate that in patients with PCOS, even if the criteria for the metabolic syndrome are not fully met, there is at least one component of the metabolic syndrome [11].

The research in the field demonstrates the presence of the risk factors for the metabolic syndrome in women with PCOS. Of these, the following appear to be important: the level of fasting insulin (which in these patients is doubled [12]) and obesity (an independent risk factor for the metabolic syndrome).

2.1.4. *Impaired glucose tolerance or type 2 diabetes mellitus*

Impaired glucose tolerance (IGT) or even type 2 diabetes mellitus (T2DM) are common in patients with PCOS with a prevalence rate of 30–40% for impaired glucose tolerance and 7.5–10% for type 2 diabetes mellitus [13, 14]. The risk of patients with PCOS to develop these pathologies is considerably higher than in healthy patients. In these cases as well obesity appears to play an important role–impaired glucose tolerance and diabetes mellitus have an increased prevalence in obese patients (31.3% IGT and 7.5% T2DM) in comparison to non-obese patients (10.3% IGT and 1.5% T2DM) suffering from PCOS.

2.1.5. *Cardiovascular disease*

It is not known exactly to what extent PCOS would be an independent risk factor for cardiovascular diseases but, unquestionably, through associated pathologies (obesity, increased resistance to insulin, IGT, T2DM, and/or dyslipidemia), it contributes to an increased risk [15].

2.2. Improvement of hyperandrogenic symptoms (hirsutism, acne, scalp hair loss)

Most experts consider that hyperandrogenism is the main characteristic of PCOS [16], whether is biochemically or clinically identified. Alteration in insulin action as well as enzymatic defaults has been discussed as possible pathogenic theories.

Studies suggest that the androgenic hyper-responsiveness that characterizes women with PCOS is probably due to the factors controlled by insulin sensitization rather than luteinizing hormone (LH), adrenocorticotropin hormone (ACTH), or ovarian steroids *per se* [16]. Multiple molecular and cellular pathways seem to be involved in the production of androgenic hormones, most of them involving ovarian theca cells, insulin receptors, Cytochrome P450 17α-monooxygenase (P450c17) activity as well as components of mitogen-activated protein kinase (MAPK) insulin pathway.

The clinical correspondence of this intricate biochemical processes have incredible impact on patients' quality of life and psychological status. Virilising signs and symptoms, acne and hirsutism are most often the first elements to lead to the clinical suspicion of PCOS.

Obesity is a key metabolic entity in some PCOS patients. Because of its undeniable influence on insulin resistance, it has become a target to treat when identified. PCOS women, who are obese tend to have higher hirsutism and acne scores than their lean counterparts [16]. The consequent importance of weight loss is therefore essential to be taken into account. It is certified in medical literature that a weight loss of 5–10% can reduce hyperandrogenism and insulin levels [17]. Lifestyle modifications reside once again as the first step therapeutical management in patients with PCOS.

2.3. Prevention of endometrial hyperplasia

The modified metabolic background associated with PCOS is basically characterized by unbalanced estrogen serum levels due to lack of progesterone production. Left untreated, the main effects of this modified environment leads to atypical endometrial hyperplasia, and endometrial dysfunction-induced infertility [18].

Even though progesterone-based oral contraceptive therapy is often efficacious [19], approximately 30% of women with PCOS fail to respond to such treatment [20] and progress to the development of atypical hyperplasia and further transformation to endometrial cancer [21].

The mechanism of progesterone resistance is determined at molecular level and based on the imbalance of two progesterone receptor (PR) isoforms PRA and PRB. Patients with PCOS have a modified ratio of PRA to PRB receptors present on stromal and epithelial cells of endometrium [21].

Progesterone resistance is associated with insulin resistance [20] and this way, a new perspective in the prevention of endometrial hyperplasia can be contoured: targeted therapy on reducing insulin resistance may benefit both endometrial tissue and serum hyperinsulinemia.

2.4. Voluntary contraception for patients

Although most of PCOS-diagnosed patients complain about the inability to pursue a pregnancy, it is important to have in mind the situation when women diagnosed and treated for PCOS do not want to obtain a pregnancy.

A recent study states that in women aged 28–33 years old, women with PCOS were less likely to be using contraception (61 versus 79%, $P < 0.001$) and more likely to be trying to conceive (56 versus 45%, $P < 0.001$), compared with women not reporting PCOS [22]. However, the same study mentions that fewer women with PCOS (61%) were using contraception than women without PCOS (79%) ($P = 0.001$) [22].

Because women with oligomenorrhea ovulate intermittently and rarely use contraception-unwanted pregnancy may occur.

2.5. Induced ovulation for patients pursuing pregnancy

As part of the PCOS, infertility secondary to anovulation is usually the main complaint of patients diagnosed with this metabolic disorder.

Pathological basis of infertility in this particular medical situation resides in the low Follicle-stimulating hormone (FSH) serum level, which is responsible for the impossibility of ovarian follicles to reach maturity due to their persistence in final growth stages.

http://dx.doi.org/10.5772/intechopen.73298

Aiming to treat this frequent cause of anovulation, there are two ways to ensure the wellbeing of the patient based on each woman's choice: evaluating the options for further contraception or starting a therapeutical plan for inducing ovulation.

With respect to the latter, inducing ovulation still remains a medical challenge in some patients with PCOS. There are a few known therapeutical approaches for achieving this: medical treatment with clomiphene citrate, tamoxifen, aromatase inhibitors, metformin, glucocorticoids, or gonadotropins or surgically management by laparoscopic ovarian drilling [23]; in vitro fertilization is also taken into consideration when all the other options failed to induce pregnancy.

3. Why are lifestyle changes and weight loss important in women with PCOS?

Taking into account the morpho-clinical picture of the patients with PCOS and common sense, lifestyle changes and weight loss would, at first glance, be effective. It seems simple that by adopting a healthy lifestyle and weight loss, as with the patients who do not suffer from this pathology, it would improve the metabolic profile, reduce the risk of diabetes mellitus, cardiovascular disease or endometrial hyperplasia. Moreover, there are studies that discuss the complete or at least partial disappearance of the symptoms [24] and PCOS phenotype after weight loss.

Studies with various degrees of evidence have been conducted in an attempt to quantify their effect in patients with PCOS. While some parameters are certainly improved, there are still others involved in a series of controversies.

3.1. Metabolic profile

An improved lifestyle will undoubtedly improve the distribution of the adipose tissue and will in most cases lead to weight loss. A weight loss of between 5 and 10% will ameliorate IGT and will decrease the prevalence of the metabolic syndrome and diabetes mellitus [25].

Research suggests that these interventions are associated with lower fasting insulin levels and insulin resistance [26], and consequently a decreased risk for metabolic syndrome, cardiovascular disease, and diabetes mellitus [27].

It has been shown that improvement of the lipid profile resulting from weight loss and lifestyle changes is nonuniform. Thus, in the case of some patients, a significant decrease in cholesterol levels will be observed while in others the change will be insignificant [24]. However, in all cases there will be a significant increase of high density lipoprotein (HDL)–cholesterol levels (thus reducing the risk of cardiovascular disease) and a decrease of triglyceride levels [24].

3.2. Hormonal profile

During the treatment, we also seek to improve the hormonal profile since PCOS being a pathology with deep hormonal implications. Unanimously, studies describe a decrease in the total testosterone level [28] and in androstenedione [29] as a result of lifestyle changes and weight loss. There is, however, controversy in terms of improving the level of SHBG and free androgen index (FAI) [29]. However, in all cases, an improvement in hirsutism will result when using the Ferriman-Gallwey (FG) score as an objective measuring method.

While the level of FSH increases as a result of lifestyle changes and weight loss, more by means of physical exercise than a result of diet [29], the level of LH does not seem to be improved by following a hygienic-dietary diet.

3.3. Reproductive potential

In PCOS treatment, we aim to restore both normal menstrual function and fertility. In some cases, there may also be a decrease in ovarian volume and a reduction in the number of follicles [30] following weight loss and lifestyle changes. Ovulatory menstrual cycles can be obtained for obese women with PCOS, even when the weight loss is relatively low [31], thus increasing considerably the chances of getting pregnant. However, not all patients equally respond to these measures even if their weight loss is similar [24]. Hollmann et al. describe an 80% improvement in ovulation rate and 29% in the pregnancy rate in the case of a 10% weight loss [32].

4. What lifestyle changes should be adopted for women with PCOS?

Although the last decades have been revolutionary in terms of understanding this pathology, its etiology is not elucidated, hence we cannot talk about the existence of a curative treatment, but rather of symptomatic treatments. The spectacular evolution in this field also refers to the many symptomatic treatments, whose efficiency, although relatively high, address each symptom in part and not the pathology as a whole. The change in lifestyle, with all the developments in the last decades, still seems the most approachable and most effective treatment method, at the same time covering a broad spectrum of symptoms.

When we talk about lifestyle changes, we refer to a healthy lifestyle that involves exercise and weight loss. Although in many cases, patients are able to lose weight and lead a healthy lifestyle for a while, the difficulty they encounter is to maintain this lifestyle and their weight in the long run.

A solution to this problem is the behavioral treatment by "Burtyn and co." designed specifically to help with this–a complex program that not only helps patients to lose weight efficiently but also to maintain their weight in the long term or even continue to lose more over time. Patients undergo this program for a period of 4–6 months under the supervision of a group of specialists: nutritionists and psychologists [33]. Patients learn how to choose healthy foods, how to ration their portions and how to get social support. After setting objective targets in terms of daily caloric intake, time spent on physical exercise and other behavioral changes, patients share in weekly or bi-weekly group sessions the obtained results. Specialists recommend patients to expect a weight loss of 0.5–1 kg per week, mentioning that the final target is a 10% decrease in weight relative to their initial weight [33]. They argue that by a comprehensive behavioral approach, patients manage to decrease 8–10 kilograms in weight and that about 80% of patients starting this program manage to complete it [34]. However, specialists mention that in the absence of weight maintenance therapy, regaining weight will be inevitable.

The National Institute of Health also recommends psychotherapeutic and social support for these patients in order to manage to maintain their weight in the long run or even to further lose weight.

4.1. What diets do we choose in order to lose weight?

Regarding the type of diet, there are no clinically relevant data to prove the efficacy of any of them in the case of patients suffering from PCOS. However, based on food principles and taking into account that a decrease in carbohydrate intake would lead to a decrease in hyperinsulinemia, which in turn would lower insulin resistance, low-carbohydrate diets would be favored. Nevertheless, a comparative study between a high protein/low carbohydrate diet (40% carbohydrate, 30% protein, and 30% fat) and a low protein/high carbohydrate diet (55% carbohydrate, 15% protein, and 30% fat) proved the same efficacy in both cases [26] in terms of weight loss, waist circumference decrease and effects on insulin sensitivity. The same study emphasizes the importance of a calorific deficit in PCOS treatment, noting that the differences in dietary compounds are relatively insignificant when comparing their effect on metabolic and reproductive improvements [26]. A meta-analysis of 48 clinical trials involving a total of 2886 patients concludes that regardless of the type of diet and macronutrient on which they are based, there will be a relatively comparative weight loss–the same thing happening with maintaining weights at follow-up for 6 months and 12 months [35]. The impact of the type of macronutrients used in the diet is still debated. What is certain is that less energy intake than energy consumption will result in a weight loss. Thus, high-level metabolic studies conclude that a caloric intake of less than 1000 kcal/day will show results in all cases, with no exception.

New diet hypothesis have emerged over the last few years, and here we want to mention the fast-paced ones, which are still under investigation and seem to be ground-breaking. Researchers believe that patients with PCOS might have significant benefits in terms of PCOS symptoms but also complications in the medium to long term if approaching this type of diets. The data we currently have on intermittent fasting diet obtained on rodent models are promising in terms of results. Thus, intermittent fasting diets, as compared to diets based on energy restriction of continued iso-energetic type, improve insulin sensitivity [36], provide protection for the cardiovascular system [37], and increase the lifespan of the rodent in the model. [38] Moreover, 3 days or more of the fasting will result in at least a 30% decrease in circulating insulin levels, glucose levels, and insulin-like growth factor 1 (IGF-1), which plays a key role in the metabolic homeostasis and changes associated with aging [39]. Current theories take into account the possibility that this type of diet can improve the symptoms of hyperandrogenism, based on the argument that improving insulin resistance would reduce compensatory hyperinsulinemia and ultimately the excess of androgen involved in the PCOS symptomatology.

Finally, we want to emphasize the importance of weight loss, pointing out the uselessness of this fact if the patients fail to maintain their long-term weight.

4.2. What is the importance of physical exercise?

Physical exercise is definitely a part of the lifestyle changes. Studies show that the type, frequency or duration of the exercise do not influence the results that patients get from it. It has been shown that regular, aerobic exercise of moderate intensity does not only contribute to weight loss and improved insulin resistance, but also improves reproductive outcomes, including ovulation and regulation of menstrual cycles. The recommendation for patients with PCOS in view of the improve reproductive and cardio metabolic outcomes is – aerobic physical activity of moderate intensity for 90 minutes per week [40].

5. What methods do we choose in order to obtain weight loss?

5.1. Pharmacological treatment for obesity

In a relatively recent past, following multiple clinical trials, medical journals supported the benefit of adding anti-obesity drugs to lifestyle changes–both in terms of maintaining weight in the long-term and reducing associated co-morbidities. Drugs such as sibutramine, orlistat, and rimonabant have been shown to be effective in improving the lipid profile, lowering blood pressure, glycosylated hemoglobin (in diabetics), and pro-inflammatory cytokine levels, thus reducing cardiovascular risk [41]. Meanwhile, it has been shown that the majority of these drugs instead of lowering cardiovascular risk have the opposite effect, which has led to their removal from the market [42].

Currently, drugs used in the treatment of obesity are–orlistat, lorcaserin, phentermine-topiramate, bupropion naltrexone, liraglutide and noradrenergic sympathomimetic drugs but there are no specific studies with patients suffering from PCOS. A list of medication used to treat obesity is shown in **Table 1**.

5.1.1. Drugs that alter fat digestion

Orlistat, being an inhibitor of pancreatic and gastric lipases, inhibits the hydrolysis of triglycerides from the diet by up to 30%, thus reducing total caloric intake [41]. Hence, weight loss is not significant using this medication only and requires a calorie-restricted regimen. The X-PERT study establishes a 3-month weight loss that exceeds 5% of the initial weight as an accurate predictor of long-term weight loss. A 12-month meta-analysis concludes that patients undergoing lifestyle changes that also associate orlistat as an adjuvant medication will lose an average of 8–10 kg over 12 months as opposed to those who associate lifestyle change with a placebo who will lose an average of 3–6 kg [43]. In addition to weight loss, it has positive effects in reducing cardiovascular risk factors due to its effects on triglyceride and LDL cholesterol [41]. Moreover, in Orlistat treatment, a better glycemic control with decreasing fasting glucose and glycosylated hemoglobin is noticed [44]. This is considered to be a relatively safe drug, with adverse effects mainly upon the intestinal tract such as increased defecation, fatty stools, and fecal urgency.

Drugs that alter fat digestion	Orlistat
Serotonin agonists	Lorcaserin
Sympathomimetic drugs	Phentermine
	Diethylpropion
	Benzphetamine
	Phendimetrazine
Antidepressants and antiepileptic drugs	Bupropion
	Venlafaxine
	Desvenlafaxine
	Topiramate
	Zonisamide
	Lamotrigine
	Ziprasidone
Diabetes drugs	Metformine
	Pramlintidine
	Exenatide
	Liraglutide
Combination drugs	Phentermine-topiramate
	Bupropion-naltrexone

Table 1. Medications used in the treatment of obesity and their classification.

5.1.2. Serotonin agonists

Lorcaserin is believed to activate serotonin 5-HT2c receptors stimulating pro-opiomelanocortin (POMC) neurons in the arcuate nucleus of the hypothalamus. Thus, it increases alpha-melanocortin stimulating hormone resulting in satiety and consequently in a decreased food intake [45]. Lorcaserin is indicated for the treatment of obesity when it is associated with at least one comorbidity such as type 2 diabetes mellitus, high blood pressure, high cholesterol or sleep apnea [46]. This is an alternative to orlistat, with similar efficacy but fewer side effects. In addition to weight loss, studies show that it lowers: blood pressure, heart rate, total cholesterol, LDL cholesterol, fasting glucose, and insulin levels.

5.1.3. Sympathomimetic drugs

Noradrenergic sympathomimetics, of which we currently find phentermine, diethylpropion, benzphetamine, and phendimetrazine, cause early satiety and reduce food cravings. Although they have increased effectiveness and their use is widespread, they are indicated for a treatment of a maximum of 12 weeks and have large potential for abuse. We must mention that all sympathomimetic drugs have side effects such as tachycardia, increased blood pressure, cause insomnia, constipation, nervousness, and dry mouth. In fact, their side effects on the cardiovascular system were those that caused the withdrawal of some drugs of this class from the market, such as sibutramine (removed from the market in 2010 [47] after it was shown to increase the risk of myocardial infarction and stroke [48]) or phenylpropanolamine (removed from the market due to association with increased risk of hemorrhagic stroke in women [49]).

5.1.4. Antidepressants and antiepileptic drugs

Antidepressants and antiepileptics can affect weight in different ways, while some lead to weight gain, others to loss. Among the drugs that lead to weight loss, we mention: bupropion, venlafaxine, desvenlafaxine, topiramate, zonisamide, lamotrigine, and ziprasidone [45].

Bupropion is an antidepressant commonly used in cases of smoking cessation, to prevent weight gain [50]. It can also be used in combination with naltrexone, although there are currently no data on an augmenting the effect of bupropion by naltrexone.

Topiramate is an antiepileptic agent that blocks neuronal voltage-dependent sodium channels, enhances gamma-aminobutyric acid (GABA) A activity and inhibits carbonic anhydrase, generating appetite suppression and satiety enhancement. Amongs its adverse effects, we mention paresthesia, somnolence, and metabolic acidosis. Studies recommend its use in combinations with other substances and not as a sole agent in the treatment of obesity.

Zonisamide is another antiepileptic with serotoninergic and dopaminergic activity, which has effect on weight loss. Randomized trials in obese patients demonstrate that zonisamide at high doses is superior to placebo, while at low doses has effects similar to placebo [51].

5.1.5. Diabetes drugs

Metformin is an anti-hyperglycemic biguanide, used in the treatment of type 2 diabetes mellitus. It reduces liver production and intestinal absorption of glucose and therefore insulin secretion. By its anti-lipolytic effect, free fatty acid concentrations and gluconeogenesis decrease [52, 53]. Numerous studies have been performed on obese patients with PCOS, who received metformin. While the first studies seemed to demonstrate its effects in terms of weight loss, decreased serum androgen levels (and implicitly hirsutism), restoration of menstrual cycles, and induction of ovulation [54], further studies concluded its ineffectiveness in treating hirsutism or increasing live birth rates, even if it is effective in increasing the ovulatory rates and pregnancy rates. Metformin is no longer used as a first-line treatment for oligomenorrhea or weight loss.

Pramlintide is a synthetic analog of human amylin whose effect in terms of weight loss is relatively modest, due to its slowing effect on gastric emptying and the reduction in postprandial blood glucose concentration it causes.

Exenatide is a long-acting synthetic peptide (GLP-1 -glucagon-like polypeptide-1-agonist receptor), the effect of which is the increased secretion of dose-dependent and glucose-dependent insulin. Its' use is avoided because of the relatively low weight loss effect in conjunction with its mode of administration by subcutaneous injection [45].

Liraglutide, like exenatide, is a GLP-1 analog with significant weight-reducing effects. Studies in obese, non-diabetic patients have shown better efficacy against placebo at normal doses and even orlistat when administered in high doses [55]. Among its adverse effects when administered at high doses are included nausea and vomiting, which may in part contribute to the weight-loss effect [55]. This drug is quite often avoided due to its route of administration (subcutaneous injection) but also due to its potential adverse effects, that although rare, they are severe (pancreatitis, renal impairment and gallbladder disease). Further, we consider important to mention that rodent studies have demonstrated the association of this drug with the increased frequency of thyroid C-cell tumors (benign and malignant), which is why it is not recommended in the case of the patients with personal or family history of medullary thyroid cancers [56].

5.1.6. Combination drugs

The combination of phentermine and topiramate is another two drug combination with good effect in terms of weight loss, being pharmacologically included in the sympathomimetic anorexia class. Being a two drug combination, it has a complex mechanism of action. Thus, phentermine, which is a sympathomimetic amine, like amphetamines, will reduce the appetite after the stimulation of the hypothalamus and the release of the norepinephrine. Topiramate also has appetite suppressing effects and causes rapid satiety. Studies show that after a 1-year administration, the effect of this combination drug on weight loss decreases, but nevertheless it seems to contribute in maintaining the weight obtained up to that point [57, 58]. Side effects of this drug include dry mouth, constipation, paresthesia, psychiatric and cognitive impairment. It is also contraindicated during pregnancy, having teratogenic effects [59].

The bupropion-naltrexone combination, though effective in weight loss, seems to have cardiovascular side effects, such as high blood pressure or tachycardia, so if it would be administered it would fail in addressing the underlying reason for initiating this therapy.

5.2. Surgical treatment of obesity–bariatric surgery

Bariatric surgery is indicated in cases of morbid obesity (BMI = 40 kg/m^2 or BMI greater than or equal to 35 kg/m^2 associated with different comorbidities). A study that enrolled obese patients who underwent bariatric surgery divided the treated patients into 3 groups; obese with PCOS, obese with hyperandrogenemia characteristics but with regular menstrual cycles and a third group with obese patients without hyperandrogenic traits. After applying the exclusion criteria, the group of patients with PCOS was studied in detail and the results were surprising. Within 12 +/− 5 months, the weight loss was of 41 +/− 9 kg, associated with the improvement of clinical and biochemical markers of hyperandrogenism. It was noted that an improvement in hirsutism had been observed and from a biochemical point of view markers such as: free testosterone, total testosterone, androstenedione and dehydroepiandrostenedione sulfate have been normalized while the level of SHBG increased. From a metabolic point of view, the improved insulin sensitivity was proved by the decrease in fasting insulin levels. With regard to the reproductive system, the restoration of regular menstrual cycles and ovulation were noticed [60].

A newer study, conducted in 2012, concludes that weight loss after bariatric surgery is not associated with significant changes in the menstrual cycle, the luteal phase length or the amount of blood lost during menstruation. A relatively modest improvement was found with respect to biochemical hyperandrogenism but without effects on the clinical markers of hyperandrogenism. Instead, an 8–9 day follicular phase shortening associated with decreased fertility, was observed. What was new in this study was the finding that patients undergoing bariatric surgery after weight loss improve their sex life [61].

6. Conclusion

We consider to be of major importance the adoption of a healthy lifestyle, composed of a hypo caloric diet and physical exercise that will generate weight loss. Unlike any other treatment, weight loss without adjuvant medication (which brings various side effects) in many cases leads to at least partial resolution of PCOS symptoms. Although in this chapter by enlarge we have approached the subject of slimming medications, we consider it important to use them only in carefully selected cases, lifestyle changes continue to be the first-line treatment.

Conflict of interest

The authors certify that they have NO affiliations with or involvement in any organization or entity with any financial interest (such as honoraria; educational grants; participation in speakers' bureaus; membership, employment, consultancies, stock ownership, or other equity interest; and expert testimony or patent-licensing arrangements), or non-financial interest (such as personal or professional relationships, affiliations, knowledge or beliefs) in the subject matter or materials discussed in this chapter.

Author details

Cringu Antoniu Ionescu[1,2*], Ina Popescu[1,2], Mihail Banacu[1,2] and Mihai Dimitriu[1,2]

*Address all correspondence to: antoniuginec@yahoo.com

1 University of Medicine and Pharmacy Carol Davila, Bucharest, Romania

2 Clinical Emergency Hospital St. Pantelimon, Bucharest, Romania

References

[1] Bozdag G, Mumusoglu S, Zengin D, Karabulut E, Yildiz BO. The prevalence and phenotypic features of polycystic ovary syndrome: A systematic review and meta-analysis. Human Reproduction. 2016 Dec;**31**(12):2841-2855

[2] Ehrmann DA. Polycystic ovary syndrome. The New England Journal of Medicine. 2005;**352**(12):1223

[3] Rebuffe-Scrive M et al. Anthropometric variables and metabolism in polycystic ovarian disease. Hormone and Metabolic Research. 1989;**21**:391-397

[4] Dumesic DA, Akopians AL, Madrigal VK, Ramirez E, Margolis DJ, Sarma MK, Thomas AM, Grogan TR, Haykal R, Schooler TA, Okeya BL, Abbott DH, Chazenbalk GD. Hyperandrogenism accompanies increased intra-abdominal fat storage in normal weight polycystic ovary syndrome women. The Journal of Clinical Endocrinology and Metabolism. 2016;**101**(11):4178 Epub 2016 Aug 29

[5] Corbould A, Dunaif A. The adipose cell lineage is not intrinsically insulin resistant in polycystic ovary syndrome. Metabolism. 2007;**56**(5):716

[6] Rosenfield RL. Clinical review: Adolescent anovulation: Maturational mechanisms and implications. The Journal of Clinical Endocrinology and Metabolism. 2013 Sep;**98**(9):3572-3583 Epub 2013 Aug 2

[7] Abate N et al. Relationships of generalized and regional adiposity to insulin sensitivity in men. The Journal of Clinical Investigation. 1995;**96**:88-98

[8] Dunaif A. Insulin resistance and the polycystic ovary syndrome: Mechanism and implications for pathogenesis. Endocrine Reviews. 1997;**18**:774-800

[9] Essah PA, Wickham EP, Nestler JE. The metabolic syndrome in polycystic ovary syndrome. Clinical Obstetrics and Gynecology. 2007 Mar;**50**(1):205-225

[10] Cattrall FR, Healy DL. Long-term metabolic, cardiovascular and neoplastic risks with polycystic ovary syndrome. Best Practice & Research. Clinical Obstetrics & Gynaecology. 2004;**18**:803-812

[11] Apridonidze T, Essah PA, Iuorno MJ, et al. Prevalence and characteristics of the metabolic syndrome in women with polycystic ovary syndrome. The Journal of Clinical Endocrinology and Metabolism. 2005;**90**:1929-1935

[12] Ehrmann DA, Liljenquist DR, Kasza K, et al. Prevalence and predictors of the metabolic syndrome in women with polycystic ovary syndrome. The Journal of Clinical Endocrinology and Metabolism. 2006;**91**:48-53

[13] Ehrmann DA et al. Prevalence of impaired glucose tolerance and diabetes in women with polycystic ovary syndrome. Diabetes Care. 1999;**22**:141-146

[14] Legro RS et al. Prevalence and predictors of risk for type 2 diabetes mellitus and impaired glucose tolerance in polycystic ovary syndrome: A prospective, controlled study in 254 affected women. The Journal of Clinical Endocrinology and Metabolism. 1999;**84**:165-169

[15] Lo JC, Feigenbaum SL, Yang J, Pressman AR, Selby JV, Go AS. Epidemiology and adverse cardiovascular risk profile of diagnosed polycystic ovary syndrome. The Journal of Clinical Endocrinology and Metabolism. 2006;**91**(4):1357

[16] Baptiste C, Battista M, Trottier A, et al. Insulin and hyperandrogenism in women with polycystic ovary syndrome. The Journal of Steroid Biochemistry and Molecular Biology. 2010 Oct;**122**(0). DOI: 10.1016/j.jsbmb.2009.12.010

[17] Moran L, Norman RJ. Understanding and managing disturbances in insulin metabolism and body weight in women with polycystic ovary syndrome. Best Practice & Research. Clinical Obstetrics & Gynaecology. 2004;**18**(5):719-736

[18] Hardiman P, Pillay OC, Atiomo W. Polycystic ovary syndrome and endometrial carcinoma. Lancet. 2003;**361**:1810-1812

[19] Vrbikova J, Cibula D. Combined oral contraceptives in the treatment of polycystic ovary syndrome. Human Reproduction Update. 2005;**11**:277-291

[20] Aghajanova L, Velarde MC, Giudice LC. Altered gene expression profiling in endometrium: Evidence for progesterone resistance. Seminars in Reproductive Medicine. 2010;**28**: 51-58

[21] Li X, Feng Y, Lin J, et al. Endometrial progesterone resistance and PCOS. Journal of Biomedical Science. 2014;**21**(1):2

[22] Joham AE, Boyle JA, Ranasinha S, et al. Contraception use and pregnancy outcomes in women with polycystic ovary syndrome: Data from the Australian longitudinal study on women's health. Human Reproduction. 2014 Apr;**29**(4):802-808

[23] Badawy A, Elnashar A. Treatment options for polycystic ovary syndrome. International Journal of Women's Health. 2011;**3**:25-35

[24] Pasquali R, Gambineri A, Cavazza C, Ibarra Gasparini D, Ciampaglia W, Cognigni GE, Pagotto U. Heterogeneity in the responsiveness to long-term lifestyle intervention and predictability in obese women with polycystic ovary syndrome. European Journal of Endocrinology. 2011 Jan;**164**(1):53-60. DOI: 10.1530/EJE-10-0692. Epub 2010 Oct 18

[25] Knowler WC, Barrett-Connor E, Fowler SE, Hamman RF, Lachin JM, Walker EA, Nathan DM, Diabetes Prevention Program Research Group. Reduction in the incidence of type 2 diabetes with lifestyle intervention or metformin. The New England Journal of Medicine. 2002 Feb 7;**346**(6):393-403

[26] Moran LJ, Noakes M, Clifton PM, Tomlinson L, Norman RJ. Dietary composition in restoring reproductive and metabolic physiology in overweight women with polycystic ovary syndrome. The Journal of Clinical Endocrinology and Metabolism. 2003;**88**:812-819

[27] Reaven GM. The insulin resistance syndrome: Definition and dietary approaches to treatment. Annual Review of Nutrition. 2005;**25**:391-406

[28] Moran LJ, Hutchison SK, Norman RJ, Teede HJ. Lifestyle changes in women with polycystic ovary syndrome (review). Cochrane Gynaecology and Fertility Group. 2011 July;**6**(7). DOI: 10.1002/14651858.CD007506.pub3

[29] Haqq L, McFarlane J, Dieberg G, Smart N. Effect of lifestyle intervention on the reproductive endocrine profile in women with polycystic ovarian syndrome: A systematic review and meta-analysis. Endocr Connect. 2014 Mar 1;**3**(1):36-46

[30] Crosignani PG, Colombo M, Vegetti W, Somigliana E, Gessati A, Ragni G. Overweight and obese anovulatory patients with polycystic ovaries: Parallel improvements in

anthropometric indices, ovarian physiology and fertility rate induced by diet. Human Reproduction. 2003;**18**(9):1928

[31] Restoration of Reproductive Potential by Lifestyle Modification in Obese Polycystic Ovary Syndrome: Role of Insulin Sensitivity and Luteinizing Hormone* Huber-Buchholz M-M, Carey DGP, Norman RJ. Reproductive Medicine Unit, University of Adelaide, Queen Elizabeth Hospital, Woodville, South Australia 5011; and the Department of Diabetes and Endocrinology, Princess Alexandra Hospital, Brisbane, Queensland 4102, Australia

[32] Hollmann M, Runnebaum B, Gerhard I. Effects of weight loss on the hormonal profile in obese, infertile women. Human Reproduction. 1996 Sep;**11**(9):1884-91

[33] Butryn ML, Webb V, Wadden TA. Behavioral treatment of obesity. The Psychiatric Clinics of North America. 2011 Dec;**34**(4):841-859

[34] Wadden TA, Butryn ML, Wilson C. Lifestyle modification for the management of obesity. Gastroenterology. 2007 May;**132**(6):2226-2238

[35] Johnston BC, Kanters S, Bandayrel K, Wu P, Naji F, Siemieniuk RA, Ball GD, Busse JW, Thorlund K, Guyatt G, Jansen JP, Mills EJ. Comparison of weight loss among named diet programs in overweight and obese adults: A meta-analysis. Journal of the American Medical Association. 2014 Sep;**312**(9):923-933

[36] Anson RM, Guo Z, de Cabo R, Iyun T, Rios M, Hagepanos A, Ingram DK, Lane MA, Mattson MP. Intermittent fasting dissociates beneficial effects of dietary restriction on glucose metabolism and neuronal resistance to injury from calorie intake. Proceedings of the National Academy of Sciences. 2003;**100**:6216-6220

[37] Mattson MP, Wan R. Beneficial effects of intermittent fasting and caloric restriction on the cardiovascular and cerebrovascular systems. The Journal of Nutritional Biochemistry. 2005;**16**:129-137

[38] Sogawa H, Kubo C. Influence of short-term repeated fasting on the longevity of female (NZB x NZW)F1 mice. Mechanisms of Ageing and Development. 2000;**115**:61-71

[39] Thankamony A, Capalbo D, Marcovecchio ML, Sleigh A, Jørgensen SW, Hill NR, Mooslehner K, Yeo GSH, Bluck L, Juul A, Vaag A, Dunger DB. Low circulating levels of IGF-1 in healthy adults are associated with reduced β-cell function, increased Intramyocellular lipid, and enhanced fat utilization during fasting. The Journal of Clinical Endocrinology and Metabolism. 2014;**99**:2198-2207

[40] AU Harrison CL, Lombard CB, Moran LJ, Teede HJ. Exercise therapy in polycystic ovary syndrome: A systematic review. Human Reproduction Update. 2011 Mar;**17**(2):171-183 Epub 2010 Sep 10

[41] Rubio MA, Gargallo M, Isabel Millan A, Moreno B. Drugs in the treatment of obesity: Sibutramine, orlistat and rimonabant. Public Health Nutrition. 2007;**10**:1200-1205

[42] Legro RS. Obesity and PCOS: Implications for diagnosis and treatment. Seminars in Reproductive Medicine. 2012 Dec;**30**(6):496-506. DOI: 10.1055/s-0032-1328878

[43] Leblanc ES, O'Connor E, Whitlock EP, Patnode CD, Kapka T. Effectiveness of primary care-relevant treatments for obesity in adults: A systematic evidence review for the U.S. preventive services task force. Annals of Internal Medicine. 2011;**155**(7):434

[44] Norris SL, Zhang X, Avenell A, Gregg E, Schmid CH, Kim C, et al. Efficacy of pharmacotherapy for weight loss in adults with type 2 diabetes mellitus: A meta-analysis. Archives of Internal Medicine. 2004;**164**:1395-1404

[45] George A, Bray MD. Obesity in Adults: Drug Therapy. https://www.uptodate.com/contents/obesity-in-adults-drug-therapy?source=search_result&search=obesity%20in%20adults&selectedTitle=3~150. (Accessed: September 1, 2017)

[46] FDA Highlights of Prescribing Information: BELVIQ (Lorchttps://www.uptodate.com/contents/obesity-in-adults-drug-therapy?source=search_result&search=obesity%20in%20adults&selectedTitle=3~150aserinhydrochloride) tablets, for oral use. http://www.accessdata.fda.gov/drugsatfda_docs/label/2012/022529lbl.pdf (Accessed: September 17, 2017)

[47] European Medicines Agency. European Medicines Agency Recommends Suspension of Marketing Authorisation for Sibutramine http://www.ema.europa.eu/ema/index.jsp?curl=pages/news_and_events/news/2010/01/news_detail_000985.sjsp&jsenabled=true (Accessed: October 1, 2017)

[48] James WP, Caterson ID, Coutinho W, Finer N, Van Gaal LF, Maggioni AP, Torp-Pedersen C, Sharma AM, Shepherd GM, Rode RA, Renz CL, SCOUT Investigators. Effect of sibutramine on cardiovascular outcomes in overweight and obese subjects. The New England Journal of Medicine. 2010;**363**(10):905

[49] Kernan WN, Viscoli CM, Brass LM, Broderick JP, Brott T, Feldmann E, Morgenstern LB, Wilterdink JL, Horwitz RI. Phenylpropanolamine and the risk of hemorrhagic stroke. The New England Journal of Medicine. 2000;**343**(25):1826

[50] Gadde KM, Parker CB, Maner LG, Wagner HR 2nd, Logue EJ, Drezner MK, Krishnan KR. Bupropion for weight loss: An investigation of efficacy and tolerability in overweight and obese women. Obesity Research. 2001;**9**(9):544

[51] Gadde KM, Kopping MF, Wagner HR 2nd, Yonish GM, Allison DB, Bray GA. Zonisamide for weight reduction in obese adults: A 1-year randomized controlled trial. Archives of Internal Medicine. 2012;**172**(20):1557

[52] Ferrannini E. The target of metformin in type 2 diabetes. The New England Journal of Medicine. 2014;**371**(16):1547

[53] Madiraju AK, Erion DM, Rahimi Y, Zhang XM, Braddock DT, Albright RA, Prigaro BJ, Wood JL, Bhanot S, MacDonald MJ, Jurczak MJ, Camporez JP, Lee HY, Cline GW, Samuel VT, Kibbey RG, Shulman GI. Metformin suppresses gluconeogenesis by inhibiting mitochondrial glycerophosphate dehydrogenase. Nature. 2014 Jun;**510**(7506):542-546 Epub 2014 May 21

[54] Singh-Franco D, Perez A, Harrington C. The effect of pramlintide acetate on glycemic control and weight in patients with type 2 diabetes mellitus and in obese patients without diabetes: A systematic review and meta-analysis. Diabetes, Obesity & Metabolism. 2011;**13**(2):169

[55] Astrup A, Rössner S, Van Gaal L, Rissanen A, Niskanen L, Al Hakim M, Madsen J, Rasmussen MF, Lean ME, NN8022-1807 Study Group. Effects of liraglutide in the treatment of obesity: A randomised, double-blind, placebo-controlled study. Lancet. 2009; **374**(9701):1606. Epub 2009 Oct 23

[56] FDA News Release. FDA Approves Weight–Management Drug Saxenda; Released 23 December 2014 – Web Address: http://www.fda.gov/NewsEvents/Newsroom/PressAnnouncements/ucm427913.htm (Accessed: September 15, 2017)

[57] Garvey WT, Ryan DH, Look M, Gadde KM, Allison DB, Peterson CA, Schwiers M, Day WW, Bowden CH. Two-year sustained weight loss and metabolic benefits with controlled-release phentermine/topiramate in obese and overweight adults (SEQUEL): A randomized, placebo-controlled, phase 3 extension study. The American Journal of Clinical Nutrition. 2012 Feb;**95**(2):297-308 Epub 2011 Dec 7

[58] Allison DB, Gadde KM, Garvey WT, Peterson CA, Schwiers ML, Najarian T, Tam PY, Troupin B, Day WW. Controlled-release phentermine/topiramate in severely obese adults: A randomized controlled trial (EQUIP). Obesity (Silver Spring). 2012 Feb;**20**(2):330-342 Epub 2011 Nov 03

[59] Héctor F. Escobar-Morreale, José I. Botella-Carretero, Francisco Á lvarez-Blasco, José Sancho, and José L. San Millán. The polycystic ovary syndrome associated with morbid obesity may resolve after weight loss induced by bariatric surgery. The Journal of Clinical Endocrinology and Metabolism. 2005 Dec;**90**(12):6364-6369. Epub 2005 Sep 27

[60] Legro RS, Dodson WC, Gnatuk CL, Estes SJ, Kunselman AR, Meadows JW, Kesner JS, Krieg EF Jr, Rogers AM, Haluck RS, Cooney RN. Effects of gastric bypass surgery on female reproductive function. The Journal of Clinical Endocrinology and Metabolism. 2012 Dec;**97**(12):4540-4548 Epub 2012 Oct 12

Chapter 5

Incretin System: New Pharmacological Target in Obese Women with Polycystic Ovary Syndrome

Mojca Jensterle Sever, Simona Ferjan and Andrej Janez

Additional information is available at the end of the chapter

http://dx.doi.org/10.5772/intechopen.70648

Abstract

Introduction: Obesity is highly prevalent in polycystic ovary syndrome (PCOS). It aggravates adverse features of the syndrome. Weight management by lifestyle intervention is often insufficient. We reviewed studies addressing the use of agents mediating through incretin system in obese PCOS.

Material and methods: Available relevant clinical trials were searched from PubMed.

Results: Intervention with glucagon-like peptide 1 (GLP-1) analogue liraglutide is associated with consistent body mass index (BMI) reduction in treatment-naive obese women with PCOS and in poor responders to metformin and lifestyle modification. We recognized metformin as a well-suited combination with liraglutide. We demonstrated that liraglutide could also improve eating behavior and fertility potential in obese PCOS. Furthermore, we challenged the potential association of variability of GLP-1 receptor genotype and interindividual differences in response to liraglutide. In addition, we introduced the original concept related to the enhancement of incretin axis through phosphodiesterase 4 (PDE4). Nevertheless, we considered dipeptidyl peptidase 4 inhibitors as an alternative pharmacological intervention in metformin intolerant patients with PCOS.

Conclusion: Agents mediating through incretin system in combination with lifestyle intervention and metformin could improve treatment outcomes in obese PCOS patients. Further studies are needed to establish the benefit/risk profile achieved by these potential new treatment strategies.

Keywords: GLP-1 receptor agonist, liraglutide, DPP4 inhibitor, weight reduction, PCOS

1. Introduction

Obesity is one of a key phenotype of polycystic ovary syndrome (PCOS). The risk for excess body weight in this population is up to 2.8 higher than in women without PCOS. About 60–70% of patients are being characterized as obese or overweight [1, 2]. The amount and distribution of fat is a major contributor to expression and severity of the syndrome [3, 4]. Obese women demonstrate more severe gynecological abnormalities and clinical and biochemical hyperandrogenism than normal weight or lean women with PCOS. Insulin resistance, glucose derangements including impaired glucose tolerance (IGT) and type 2 diabetes mellitus (T2DM) and an increased overall cardiovascular risk are also more likely in obese PCOS [5–7]. Weight reduction is substantial for improvement of metabolic and androgen profile, reproductive function and reducing cardiovascular risk. Weight management by lifestyle intervention often remains unsatisfactory and nonsustainable. In the present chapter, we revised limited studies addressing the potential use of agents mediating through glucagon-like peptide 1 (GLP-1) in obese PCOS. We mainly focused on the available clinical trials of GLP-1 receptor agonists in this population. In addition, we challenged the original concept related to the enhancement of GLP-1–mediated action through phosphodiesterase 4 (PDE4). Nevertheless, we considered dipeptidyl peptidase 4 inhibitors as an alternative pharmacological intervention in subgroups of PCOS with high metabolic risk.

2. Main body

2.1. Gut-brain axis in controlling eating behavior

An inability to control eating behavior is the main culprit for eating beyond metabolic needs that result in obesity. Eating behavior is a complex pattern based on communication between specific regulatory and hedonistic centers in hypothalamus and peripheral signals from gastrointestinal tract. The latter system consists of gastric emptying/distention signals and gastrointestinal regulatory (orexigenic and anorexigenic) hormones. In addition, eating behavior is regulated also by cognitive functions and emotional inputs [8, 9].

Orexigenic hormone increases before meal and stimulates hunger and food intake. The most potent known orexigenic hormone ghrelin is released from specific endocrine cells in the stomach and stimulates food intake. On the opposite, hormones, such as cholecystokinin (CCK), peptide tyrosine-tyrosine (PYY) and glucagon-like polipeptide-1 (GLP-1), produce anorexigenic signals and affect peripheral organs and centers in the central nervous system (CNS) in order to stop feeding [8].

Reports about eating behavior in PCOS population are few and the results are not conclusive. It has not been established whether eating behavior is different in obese women with PCOS when compared to weight-matched non-PCOS controls. An increased food intake was reported in animal models and clinical studies with women with PCOS when compared to healthy controls [10–14]. Furthermore, bulimia was associated with an increased frequency of PCOS, suggesting that androgens have appetite-stimulating effects and could impair the impulse control of eating behavior [15]. Disturbed appetite was also associated with altered opioid function demonstrated in PCOS linked to the stimulation of food intake and appetite for high fat/high glucose food through hedonistic centers in hypothalamus [16]. In addition, there are some evidences that disturbed regulation of gastrointestinal signals, in particular incretins, are intrinsic to PCOS [15, 17–21].

2.2. Incretin hormones

Incretins are glucagon-like peptide 1 (GLP-1) and glucose-dependent insulinotropic polypeptide (GIP). They are polypeptide gut hormones secreted from endocrine cells in the small intestine under the influence of food intake and are responsible for 50–70% of postprandial insulin secretion. This is so-called incretin effect and is proportional to the current glycemia [8, 22].

GLP-1 is produced by L cells in distal intestine. It influences glucose hemostasis after food ingestion by insulin secretion and concurrent inhibition of glucagon release. GLP-1 is involved in the regulatory mechanisms of eating behavior with direct inhibitory effect on the homeostatic and hedonic centers of appetite in the central nervous system and indirect inhibitory effect on gastric emptying rates and gastrointestinal tract motility, which result in decreased food intake and consequently in body weight reduction [8, 23].

GIP is produced by K cells, which are located in the upper small intestine. It increases glucose-dependent insulin release and has protective effect on beta cell. GIP also increases lipogenesis and has bone protective and neuroprotective effect. In contrast to GLP1, no additional effects on appetite and body weight are shown with GIP [22].

Both incretin hormones have a short half-life. They are rapidly inactivated by the enzyme dipeptidyl peptidase 4 (DPP4).

Obesity with the onset of insulin resistance and consequent metabolic diseases, such as impaired glucose tolerance and type 2 diabetes, impairs the effect of incretins. Postprandial GLP-1 concentration in obese people is lower than in people with normal body weight [24–27]. Similarly, lower postprandial GLP-1 values were measured in patients with type 2 diabetes, while the GIP response in this population was preserved [28–32].

2.3. Incretin hormones in PCOS

Current reports about GLP-1 secretion in PCOS are not consistent. Some studies found similar fasting GLP-1 levels in PCOS compared with age- and BMI-matched controls [21, 33–35], whereas others reported decreased or increased fasting levels of GLP-1 in PCOS [36, 37]. Regarding postprandial levels of GLP-1, some authors demonstrated that postprandial plasma levels of GLP-1 did not differ between subjects with and without PCOS [20, 34, 35]. On the other hand, another study demonstrated lower GLP-1 levels in PCOS at the end of oral glucose tolerance test (OGTT) compared to the control group, whereas fasting GLP-1 levels did not differ between two groups [21]. However, lower fasting GLP-1 levels and a weakened GLP-1 response to standardized mixed meal in women with PCOS versus healthy control group were also reported [37]. Contrary, another group found higher fasting GLP-1 levels in PCOS patients; while at the end of OGTT, GLP-1 levels did not differ between groups [36].

Also studies concerning the GLP-1 response in PCOS patients in relation to body weight are not conclusive. Some authors demonstrated no difference in GLP-1 between lean and obese patients with PCOS during OGTT, whereas others reported lower levels of GLP-1 in obese PCOS patients compared to lean age-matched PCOS patients and healthy lean controls [20].

There are only few studies evaluating GIP levels in women with PCOS. Compared with BMI- and age-matched controls, most of them demonstrated no difference in fasting GIP levels [20, 33–35, 38], yet some have found increased fasting GIP [21]. The results of postprandial GIP levels in PCOS compared to matched controls are more inconsistent. While some studies did not find differences in GIP levels [34], other found increased [21, 38] or decreased [20, 35] GIP levels after OGTT.

2.4. Therapeutic interventions targeting incretin system in obese PCOS

Weight reduction is substantial for improvement of hyperandrogenism and reproductive function in obese women with PCOS [4, 39]. Furthermore, weight loss has beneficial effects on all cardiovascular risk factors, including glycemic control, hypertension and hyperlipidemia in this population [39–41].

2.4.1. Lifestyle intervention in PCOS

Recent clinical practice guidelines recommend lifestyle modification as the first-line intervention in obese PCOS [42]. Low glucose index diet and hypocaloric diet lead to decrease in body mass index (BMI), waist circumference and waist-to-hip ratio [39]. Modification of lifestyle is associated with an important reduction in testosterone and an increase in serum sex hormone-binding globulin (SHBG) levels, leading to reduced free androgen index [43–45]. Furthermore, beneficial effect of appropriate lifestyle on metabolic abnormalities, such as a decrease in serum insulin and fasting glucose levels, an improvement in insulin resistance (IR) and decline in diastolic blood pressure, is known [43–45]. Lifestyle changes also lead to improvement of fertility function [39, 46, 47]. Two small studies in PCOS proved the impact of dietary intervention on ghrelin, whereas no studies evaluated the impact of lifestyle intervention on incretin hormones in this population [17, 48]. However, the treatment goals with lifestyle intervention are usually hardly achievable and nonsustainable in everyday life.

2.4.2. Metformin in PCOS

Metformin as an established treatment in PCOS with many potential roles, including attenuating IR and direct blocking ovarian androgen production, has inconsistently demonstrated weight reduction. The absolute weight loss that was best documented in obese rather in lean women with PCOS had been about 2.7 kg, representing less than 5% of weight reduction

[49, 50]. No benefit regarding weight reduction was recognized when metformin was added on lifestyle changes. In a small study with 19 lean and 21 obese PCOS patients, the impact of metformin on incretin hormones was demonstrated with the increase of GLP-1 during OGTT with 8-month metformin intervention [35].

2.4.3. GLP-1 receptor agonists in PCOS

The available recent data offer new opportunity to include an adjunct management in obese PCOS patients who have not responded to lifestyle modification with or without metformin [51, 52].

GLP-1 receptor agonists (GLP-1 RA) are class of antidiabetes medications, which are incretin mimetics. There are six GLP-1 RAs approved and available, of which only liraglutide and exenatide have been studied in PCOS [53–61]. Studies have been of short duration and have all shown the expected effective weight reduction with GLP-1Ras alone or in combination with metformin and improvement in glucose parameters with variable results on gynecological abnormalities and hyperandrogenism (**Table 1**).

2.4.3.1. Liraglutide in PCOS

Liraglutide is a long-acting GLP-1 RA analogue that is 97% homologous to human GLP-1. Its dose-dependent effect on weight loss was first observed in overweight patients with type 2 diabetes and later also in overweight subjects without diabetes. In dose of 3 mg, it was recently approved for weight management in many countries [62–65].

Study	Weight reduction	Improved eating behavior	Decreased insulin resistance	Decreased fasting and/ or post-load glucose level	Reduced hyperandrogenism	Improved menstrual frequency
Elkind-Hirsch et al. [59]	x		x	x	x	x
Rasmussen and Lindenberg [55]	x					/
Kahal et al. [58]	x		/		/	
Jensterle Sever et al. [53]	x		/	x	/	/
Jensterle et al. [60]	x		x	x	/	x
Jensterle et al. [56]	x	x				
Jensterle et al. [57]	x		x	x	x	
Nylander et al. [61]	x				x	x

Note: x = yes; / = no effect.

Table 1. Reported effects of GLP-1 agonist treatment in women with PCOS.

The efficacy of 3 mg liraglutide on weight loss was studied in a Satiety and Clinical Adiposity-Liraglutide Evidence (SCALE) series of four trials involving 5358 patients who were divided in different patient categories. SCALE-prediabetes involved 3731 adult patients with prediabetes and BMI ≥ 30 kg/m^2 or BMI ≥ 27 kg/m^2 and associated hypertension or dyslipidemia [66]. SCALE-diabetes involved 846 adult patients with type 2 diabetes and BMI kg/m^2 ≥ 27 who were on peroral hypoglycemic therapy [63]. In SCALE Maintenance trial, the ability of high-dose liraglutide to maintain weight lost following a low-calorie diet and exercise intervention was observed on 422 obese nondiabetic patients [67]. SCALE OSA involved 359 nondiabetic obese adults with moderate or severe obstructive sleep apnea, who were unable to use CPAP [68]. In composite data analysis of the SCALE clinical trials, liraglutide 3.0 mg led to 7.5% weight loss over 1 year.

Its impact on weight loss appears to be due to reduction of appetite, mediated partly through incretin effect and consequent suppress of ghrelin release and partly through its influence on gastric emptying via the autonomous nervous system [69]. Liraglutide is the only known glucose-lowering agent with proven ability to regulate eating behavior. It probably sufficiently activates mesolimbic GLP-1 receptor and suppresses hunger-driven feeding and reduces the hedonic value of food and food motivation [69]. It was demonstrated that liraglutide produces significant improvements in eating behavior in obese patients with T2DM and importantly reduces lust for fat intake. The effect was sustained 6 months after withdrawal of liraglutide [70, 71].

Current data about liraglutide use in obese patients with PCOS are very limited. In a 12-week study with 40 obese PCOS women who had been insufficiently treated with lifestyle modification and metformin regarding weight reduction, liraglutide 1.2 mg sc QD alone or in combination with metformin 1000 mg BID was associated with significantly greater weight loss when compared to metformin monotherapy. The mean weight loss in combined treatment was 6.5 kg. Liraglutide monotherapy resulted in 3.8 kg loss and metformin alone in 1.2 kg loss. The majority of patients who achieved at least 5% of weight reduction were on combination therapy. Two-hour post-load glucose level was significantly lower in the treatment groups with liraglutide. Menstrual frequency and androgen profile were not significantly changed in any group over the observed period [53]. Another study with newly diagnosed obese PCOS patients with high metabolic risk also showed significantly greater weight reduction with liraglutide therapy when compared to metformin and lifestyle intervention [54]. In both studies, liraglutide 1.2 mg QD was used before liraglutide in a dose of 3 mg was approved as an anti-obesity drug. In an observational study of 84 overweight and obese women with PCOS with mean duration of 27.8 weeks and with liraglutide doses ranging from 0.6 mg up to 1.8 mg per day, combined treatment with liraglutide and metformin was associated with significant weight reduction of 9 kg. More than 80% of patients lost at least 5% of baseline weight [55]. It was also reported that liraglutide treatment improved the impaired eating behavior of women with PCOS who were pre-treated with metformin and switched to liraglutide for 12 weeks. There was significant decrease in emotional eating that correlated with weight loss [56].

Adding metformin to liraglutide was proven as well-suited combination that enhances the therapeutic index of GLP-1RA and enables the use of lower liraglutide dose [57, 72–75]. Metformin in combination with low dose liraglutide 1.2 mg was superior to low dose liraglutide 1.2 mg alone in reducing weight after 12 weeks in treatment naïve obese women with PCOS. Participants on combined treatment achieved clinically meaningful ≥5% weight loss in almost 60% compared to about 40% of good responders with low dose liraglutide monotherapy. Androgens were lower in all patients at study completion, yet only androstenedione was significantly decreased in the combination group. Systolic blood pressure was significantly lowered in the liraglutide arm. All subjects demonstrated a significant improvement in insulin resistance and fasting and 2-hour post-load glucose level [57]. The observed benefits of GLP-1 RAs in combination with metformin are mechanistically well supported. In animal models and in humans with or without type 2 diabetes, administration of metformin led to increase in GLP-1 concentration [74, 75]. It directly stimulated GLP-1 production and secretion from L cells through crosstalk between the insulin and Wnt signaling pathways. In addition, its impact on alteration in bile acid absorption may result in increased GLP-1 secretion. Furthermore, it was demonstrated that metformin enhances expression of GLP1 receptors through a mechanism requiring PPAR-alpha [72]. It also has a small impact on the inhibition of DPP4 activity [76].

Another interesting avenue was opened with a study conducted with 57 women with PCOS received liraglutide for 12 weeks. Recognizing that the weight reducing effects of GLP-1 RAs are mediated through GLP-1 receptor, it was hypothesized that inter-individual difference in weight loss potential of liraglutide might be linked with genetic variability of GLP-1 receptor. It was demonstrated that a difference in a liraglutide-induced weight loss potential in phenotypically and metabolically homogeneous group of obese women with PCOS was based on some GLP1-R genotype [77].

The majority of available studies with liraglutide in PCOS did not focus on the cardiometabolic endpoints. In a small study, the potential impact of liraglutide on markers of liver fibrosis in PCOS was primarily investigated. Liraglutide was found to reduce procollagen type 3 amino terminal peptide, a predictor of liver cirrhosis. An average weight reduction of 3.0 kg achieved with larger dosage of 1.8 mg sc QD in monotherapy was observed over 24 weeks [78]. In another study, 6-month intervention with liraglutide was associated with significant reduction in atherothrombosis markers, including inflammation, endothelial function and clotting. The positive effect equally affected young obese women with PCOS and controls [58].

Few studies suggested an increase in menstrual frequencies when taking GLP-1 RAs [59–61]. The most recent study reported that liraglutide improved bleeding ratio and decreased ovarian volume with liraglutide when compared to placebo [61]. Moreover, after liraglutide discontinuation, one small 12-week study conducted with 40 infertile PCOS reported an increase of fertility potential. Women were randomized into three groups: MET group was treated with metformin 1000 mg BID, COMBI group was on combined treatment with metformin 1000 mg BID and liraglutide 1.2 mg QD and CON group were controls. CON directly proceeded with ovarian stimulation protocol, whereas MET and COMBI started with stimulation after 4-week washout period. More than 5% of weight reduction was achieved in over 75% in COMBI and about 45% of patients in metformin arm. In high responders who lost more than 5% of body weight, numbers of blastocysts/patient were greater in both treatment arms than in CON. High responders in COMBI had the highest number of oocytes/patient and of mature oocyte. In COMBI 3, patients became spontaneously pregnant before IVF in medication-free period. The high rate of spontaneous pregnancies in COMBI after liraglutide discontinuation implies the potential role of GLP-1 in reproduction in the pre-conception period [79]. In line with these preliminary results, new data support a role for GLP-1RAs in fertility beyond merely weight reduction [51]. In animal models, GLP-1 and GLP receptors have been identified directly in the hypothalamo-pituitary ovary axis [80].

2.4.3.2. Exenatide in PCOS

The single report evaluating the effect of short-acting GLP-1 RA exenatide in PCOS was a 24-week randomized study demonstrated a mean weight loss of 3.2 kg with exenatide monotherapy in a dose of 10 μg twice daily, 6.0 kg with exenatide in adjunct to metformin and 1.6 kg with metformin alone. Combined therapy was superior to either monotherapy in improving menstrual frequency and ovulation rate. The ovulation rate was 86% in the combined group compared to 50% in exenatide monotherapy and 29% in metformin alone group. IR and insulin sensitivity were improved in all groups. Total cholesterol and triglyceride decreased with combined therapy compared to metformin alone [59]. Weight reductions with exenatide were of comparable magnitude to the liraglutide effect in PCOS, but achieved in a longer period of time with a larger drop out [53, 59]. The study with exenatide was the first study addressing intervention with GLP-1 Ras in PCOS population.

2.4.3.3. Safety profile of GLP-RAs in PCOS

GLP1Ras appear to be well tolerated in PCOS population. The main side effect was nausea, which was transient and did not result in study withdrawals. In studies when GLP-1RA liraglutide was dosed at 1.2 mg (the middle dose for diabetes therapy) and combined with metformin in maximum dose (1 g BID), nausea appeared to be less common, which may be due to the lower doses of liraglutide administered [57, 60]. So far, there is no safety data about GLP-1RA use in pregnancy. They are generally classified as pregnancy class C. Therefore, the use of these medications in this population would require use of contraception while on therapy. Counseling women who are planning pregnancy would include a washout period.

2.4.4. PDE4 inhibitors in PCOS

Less recognized and completely distinct regulatory mechanisms related to the enhancement of GLP-1–mediated action represent an inhibition of phosphodiesterase (PDE) 4. The first drug specifically targeting PDE4 was roflumilast. It was approved for treatment of chronic inflammatory diseases, primarily chronic obstructive pulmonary disease (COPD), due to its efficient anti-inflammatory effect [81]. Collaterally, 1-year treatment of COPD with roflumilast was associated with a weight loss of about 2 kg within 12 months [81]. Beneficial effect of roflumilast on metabolic parameters and glucose homeostasis accompanied with mean weight reduction of approximately 2 kg versus placebo was also demonstrated with a short-term use of roflumilast in newly diagnosed T2DM without COPD [82]. A small randomized study with obese PCOS women demonstrated that treatment with roflumilast 500 mg per day in combination with metformin 1000 mg twice per day significantly reduced body weight in obese PCOS when compared to metformin monotherapy. Weight loss was primarily due to visceral fat mass reduction with the between treatment difference of about 5 kg [83]. These observations gave rise to the hypothesis that PDE4 is involved in regulation of signaling pathways linked to GLP-1 release [84]. In line with this consideration are data from experimental rodent model where a single treatment with roflumilast enhanced plasma GLP-1 levels up to 2.5-fold [84]. A direct comparison of short-term intervention with liraglutide and roflumilast addressing weight management was performed in PCOS-related obesity [60]. It was demonstrated that both monotherapy with liraglutide and roflumilast were associated with significant weight reduction in obese PCOS when compared to metformin monotherapy. Reduction of weight with liraglutide was greater than with roflumilast [60].

2.4.5. *DPP4 inhibitors in PCOS*

The endogenous incretins are quickly degraded by DPP4 in serum. Degradation of endogenous incretins can be prevented by DPP4 inhibitors. DPP4 inhibitors are taken orally and are used as antidiabetic agents. They influence glucose homeostasis through the enhancement of endogenous incretion hormones. As incretin enhances insulin secretion in response to meal, DPP4 inhibitors do not cause hypoglycemia. They have been reported to cause a 0.5–1% HbA1c reduction [85, 86]. Five DPP4 inhibitors are approved in the treatment of type 2 diabetes: sitagliptin, alogliptin, saxagliptin, vildagliptin and linagliptin. The role of enhancement of endogenous GLP-1 with DPP4 inhibitors in the treatment of obese PCOS patient is yet to be established. So far, only sitagliptin, alogliptin and saxagliptin were studied in PCOS (**Table 2**).

The present evidences suggest that DPP4 inhibitors preserve beta cell function [23, 87]. The fact that body weight gain and associated insulin resistance lead to increased load of beta cells and consequent beta cell dysfunction give rise to thoughts that the use of DPP4 inhibitors in treatment of PCOS with high metabolic risk is reasonable.

Another aspect is weight management. The enhancement of endogenous incretin hormones by DPP4 inhibitors is generally described as being weight neutral, although modest weight reduction has been seen in some clinical trials, particularly when DPP4 inhibitors are used

Study	DPP4 inhibitor	Beta cell function	Insulin sensitivity	Insulin resistance	T2DM development	Weight
Jensterle et al. [92]	Alogliptin	Improved	Increased	Decreased		
Ferjan et al. [93]	Sitagliptin	Improved			Decreased	Less weight gain compared to lifestyle
Elkind-Hirsch et al. [94]	Saxagliptin	Improved	Increased	Decreased	Decreased	Reduction
Jensterle Sever et al. [95]	Sitagliptin					In combination with metformin less weight gain compared to metformin monotherapy

Table 2. Reported effects of treatment with DPP4 inhibitors in women with PCOS.

in combination with metformin [88, 89]. Nevertheless, the mere fact that DPP4 inhibition is not associated with the weight gain that typically accompanies improved glycemic control in patients with T2DM suggests that DPP4 inhibitors may not be completely neutral in this respect [90]. Slowing of gastric emptying that might reinforce the sustained change of eating behavior was also demonstrated with treatment with DPP4 inhibitor sitagliptin [91].

The first study addressing the preservation of beta cell function in PCOS with DPP4 inhibitor reported an increase of insulin sensitivity and significant decrease of insulin resistance when alogliptin was added to metformin. Even greater improvement of these parameters was seen when triplet therapy with alogliptin, pioglitazone and metformin was used [92]. Beneficial effects of another DPP4 inhibitor sitagliptin were recently reported in metformin intolerant women with PCOS and high metabolic risk. After metformin withdrawal, a 12-week treatment with sitagliptin leads to significant improvement in beta cell function and prevented conversion rate from normal to impaired glucose tolerance and type 2 diabetes when compared to placebo [93]. Preliminary data suggest that DPP4 inhibitors seem to be a promising alternative in PCOS women with high metabolic risk who have failed with lifestyle intervention and are metformin intolerant. Future larger designs of longer duration should be powered.

A small single blind, randomized study on prediabetic PCOS women reported beneficial effect of DPP4 inhibitor saxagliptin on glucose homeostasis, metabolic parameters and clinical status. A 16-week intervention with saxagliptin/metformin (5 mg/2000 mg), monotherapy with saxagliptin (5 mg) and monotherapy with metformin (2000 mg) lead to normalization in glucose homeostasis in 91, 55 and 25% of patients, respectively. Improvement of metabolic parameters and clinical status was reported in all groups [94].

In a recent randomized study, another potential use of DPP4 inhibitors was demonstrated. Enhancement of endogenous GLP-1 signaling by sitagliptin prevented the expected weight regain after liraglutide 3.0 mg cessation in women with PCOS. During a 12-week follow-up period, sitagliptin in adjunct to metformin resulted in weight maintenance, whereas a switch to metformin alone resulted in a significant weight regain after liraglutide discontinuation. It was also demonstrated that the ability to resist emotional eating was greater in combined treatment than in monotherapy with metformin [95]. The observation provides first clinical findings suggesting that DPP4 inhibition may prevent weight regain after liraglutide cessation. This sequential treatment concept is particularly useful in patients who became intolerant, develop treatment resistance or decide to stop the antiobesity treatment with liraglutide. Further research is necessary to fully understand the cross talks between effects of peripheral signals of endogenous GLP-1 and central areas of satiety and reward in obese subjects.

2.4.6. Bariatric surgery in PCOS

Bariatric surgery is a well-established and effective method for the treatment of extreme obesity for well-informed and motivated patients with a BMI > 40 kg/m^2 or >35 kg/m^2, with at least one comorbidity related to obesity and who have been previously unsuccessful with medical treatment for obesity [96]. The mechanism of weight loss induced by bariatric surgery is multifactorial. Beside reduced gastric volume [97, 98], weight reduction could be possibly explained with the changes in gut-brain axis. Gastrointestinal bypass surgery results in a quick delivery of nutrients to the small intestine associated with large increase in postprandial levels of GLP1 and PYY hormones

[97–100]. Nevertheless, the mere fact that postoperative weight loss was significantly correlated to the magnitude of GLP1 response (57 Holst) suggests that GLP1 has major role in weight balance.

There is currently no clear consensus on the role of bariatric surgery in the treatment of obese patients with PCOS. Studies in PCOS are very heterogeneous with a small number of patients. Beneficial observations were reported after laparoscopic Roux-en-Y gastric band (RYGB) operation, in two small studies, where post-operational weight loss was associated with resolution of hirsutism in 29–52% of patients, resolution of type 2 diabetes, improvement of hypertension and dyslipidemia was also reported. Moreover, in both studies, significant improvement in conception rate was observed [101, 102]. The same effects were also reported in small studies on obese PCOS patients who underwent gastric banding, gastric plication and laparoscopic sleeve gastrectomy [103, 104].

3. Conclusion

Agents mediating through GLP-1 effects in combination with lifestyle intervention and metformin could potentially improve treatment outcomes in obese PCOS via co-targeting multifactorial origin of obesity and concomitant abnormalities intrinsically related to PCOS. Based on the limited available data, GLP-1RAs, in particular liraglutide, should be considered in obese PCOS. Enhanced understanding of the direct impact on GLP-1 beyond weight reducing and metabolic effects at the levels of pituitary and ovary are expected within the next 5 years [51]. Larger and longer randomized studies are needed to establish metabolic, reproductive and cardiovascular risk reduction and assess sustainability and safety profile of the benefits achieved by these potential new treatment strategies.

Author details

Mojca Jensterle Sever*, Simona Ferjan and Andrej Janez

*Address all correspondence to: mojca.jensterlesever@kclj.si

Department of Endocrinology, Diabetes and Metabolic Diseases, University Medical Centre Ljubljana, Slovenia

References

[1] Lim SS, Davies MJ, Norman RJ, Moran LJ. Overweight, obesity and central obesity in women with polycystic ovary syndrome: A systematic review and meta-analysis. Human Reproduction Update. 2012;**18**(6):618-637. DOI: 10.1093/humupd/dms030

[2] De Leo V, la Marca A, Petraglia F. Insulin-lowering agents in the management of polycystic ovary syndrome. Endocrine Reviews. 2003;**24**(5):633-667. DOI: 10.1210/er.2002-0015

[3] Lass N, Kleber M, Winkel K, Wunsch R, Reinehr T. Effect of lifestyle intervention on features of polycystic ovarian syndrome, metabolic syndrome, and intima-media thickness in obese adolescent girls. The Journal of Clinical Endocrinology and Metabolism. 2011;**96**(11):3533-3540. DOI: 10.1210/jc.2011-1609

[4] Crosignani PG, Colombo M, Vegetti W, Somigliana E, Gessati A, Ragni G. Overweight and obese anovulatory patients with polycystic ovaries: Parallel improvements in anthropometric indices, ovarian physiology and fertility rate induced by diet. Human Reproduction (Oxford, England). 2003;**18**(9):1928-1932. DOI: 10.1093/humrep/deg367

[5] Moran LJ, Misso ML, Wild RA, Norman RJ. Impaired glucose tolerance, type 2 diabetes and metabolic syndrome in polycystic ovary syndrome: A systematic review and meta-analysis. Human Reproduction Update. 2010;**16**(4):347-363. DOI: 10.1093/humupd/dmq001

[6] Elting MW, Korsen TJ, Bezemer PD, Schoemaker J. Prevalence of diabetes mellitus, hypertension and cardiac complaints in a follow-up study of a Dutch PCOS population. Human Reproduction (Oxford, England). 2001;**16**(3):556-560. DOI: 10.1093/humrep/16.3.556

[7] Legro RS, Kunselman AR, Dodson WC, Dunaif A. Prevalence and predictors of risk for type 2 diabetes mellitus and impaired glucose tolerance in polycystic ovary syndrome: A prospective, controlled study in 254 affected women. The Journal of Clinical Endocrinology and Metabolism. 1999;**84**(1):165-169. DOI: 10.1210/jc.84.1.165

[8] Woods SC, D'Alessio DA. Central control of body weight and appetite. The Journal of Clinical Endocrinology and Metabolism. 2008;**93**(11 Suppl 1):S37-S50. DOI: 10.1210/jc.2008-1630

[9] Saydam BO, Yildiz BO. Gut-brain axis and metabolism in polycystic ovary syndrome. Current Pharmaceutical Design. 2016;**22**:1-16. DOI: 10.2174/1381612822666160715

[10] Douglas CC, Norris LE, Oster RA, Darnell BE, Azziz R, Gower BA. Difference in dietary intake between women with polycystic ovary syndrome and healthy controls. Fertility and Sterility. 2006;**86**(2):411-417. DOI: 10.1016/j.fertnstert.2005.12.054

[11] Zhang J, Liu Y, Liu X, Xu L, Zhou L, Tang L, et al. High intake of energy and fat in Southwest Chinese women with PCOS: A population-based case-control study. PLoS One. 2015;**10**(5):e0127094. DOI: 10.1371/journal.pone.0127094

[12] Ahmadi A, Akbarzadeh M, Mohammadi F, Akbari M, Jafari B, Tolide-Ie HR. Anthropometric characteristics and dietary pattern of women with polycystic ovary syndrome. Indian Journal of Endocrinology and Metabolism. 2013;**17**(4):672-676. DOI: 10.4103/2230-8210.113759

[13] Graff SK, Mário FM, Alves BC, Spritzer PM. Dietary glycemic index is associated with less favorable anthropometric and metabolic profiles in polycystic ovary syndrome women with different phenotypes. Fertility and Sterility. 2013;**100**(4):1081-1088. DOI: 10.1016/j.fertnstert.2013.06.005

[14] Moran LJ, Ranasinha S, Zoungas S, McNaughton SA, Brown WJ, Teede HJ. The contribution of diet, physical activity and sedentary behaviour to body mass index in women with and without polycystic ovary syndrome. Human Reproduction (Oxford, England). 2013;**28**(8):2276-2283. DOI: 10.1093/humrep/det256

[15] Naessén S, Carlström K, Garoff L, Glant R, Hirschberg AL. Polycystic ovary syndrome in bulimic women—An evaluation based on the new diagnostic criteria. Gynecological Endocrinology: The Official Journal of the International Society of Gynecological Endocrinology. 2006;**22**(7):388-394. DOI: 10.1080/09513590600847421

[16] Berent-Spillson A, Love T, Pop-Busui R, Sowers M, Persad CC, Pennington KP, et al. Insulin resistance influences central opioid activity in polycystic ovary syndrome. Fertility and Sterility. 2011;**95**(8):2494-2498. DOI: 10.1016/j.fertnstert.2011.03.031

[17] Moran LJ, Noakes M, Clifton PM, Wittert GA, Tomlinson L, Galletly C, et al. Ghrelin and measures of satiety are altered in polycystic ovary syndrome but not differentially affected by diet composition. The Journal of Clinical Endocrinology and Metabolism. 2004;**89**(7):3337-3344. DOI: 10.1210/jc.2003-031583

[18] Moran LJ, Noakes M, Clifton PM, Wittert GA, Roux CWL, Ghatei MA, et al. Postprandial ghrelin, cholecystokinin, peptide YY, and appetite before and after weight loss in overweight women with and without polycystic ovary syndrome. The American Journal of Clinical Nutrition. 2007;**86**(6):1603-1610

[19] Daghestani MH, Daghestani MH, El-Mazny A. Circulating ghrelin levels and the polycystic ovary syndrome: Correlation with the clinical, hormonal and metabolic features. European Journal of Obstetrics, Gynecology, and Reproductive Biology. 2011;**155**(1):65-68. DOI: 10.1016/j.ejogrb.2010.11.019

[20] Pontikis C, Yavropoulou MP, Toulis KA, Kotsa K, Kazakos K, Papazisi A, et al. The incretin effect and secretion in obese and lean women with polycystic ovary syndrome: A pilot study. Journal of Women's Health (2002). 2011;**20**(6):971-976. DOI: 10.1089/jwh.2010.2272

[21] Vrbikova J, Hill M, Bendlova B, Grimmichova T, Dvorakova K, Vondra K, et al. Incretin levels in polycystic ovary syndrome. European Journal of Endocrinology. 2008;**159**(2):121-127. DOI: 10.1530/EJE-08-0097

[22] Phillips LK, Prins JB. Update on incretin hormones. Annals of the New York Academy of Sciences. 2011;**1243**:E55-E74. DOI: 10.1111/j.1749-6632.2012.06491.x

[23] Garber AJ. Incretin therapy – Present and future. The Review of Diabetic Studies: RDS. 2011;**8**(3):307-322. DOI: 10.1900/RDS.2011.8.307

[24] Hussein MS, Abushady MM, Refaat S, Ibrahim R. Plasma level of glucagon-like peptide 1 in obese Egyptians with normal and impaired glucose tolerance. Archives of Medical Research. 2014;**45**(1):58-62. DOI: 10.1016/j.arcmed.2013.10.012

[25] de Luis DA, Aller R, Conde R, Primo D, Izaola O, Castro MJ, et al. Basal glucagon-like peptide 1 levels and metabolic syndrome in obese patients. Journal of Investigative Medicine: The Official Publication of the American Federation for Clinical Research. 2012;**60**(6):874-877. DOI: 10.2310/JIM.0b013e3182544f9e

[26] Carr RD, Larsen MO, Jelic K, Lindgren O, Vikman J, Holst JJ, et al. Secretion and dipeptidyl peptidase-4-mediated metabolism of incretin hormones after a mixed meal or glucose ingestion in obese compared to lean, nondiabetic men. The Journal of Clinical Endocrinology and Metabolism. 2010;**95**(2):872-878. DOI: 10.1210/jc.2009-2054

[27] Muscelli E, Mari A, Casolaro A, Camastra S, Seghieri G, Gastaldelli A, et al. Separate impact of obesity and glucose tolerance on the incretin effect in normal subjects and type 2 diabetic patients. Diabetes. 2008;**57**(5):1340-1348. DOI: 10.2337/db07-1315

[28] Nauck M, Stöckmann F, Ebert R, Creutzfeldt W. Reduced incretin effect in Type 2 (non-insulin-dependent) diabetes. Diabetologia. 1986;**29**(1):46-52. DOI: 10.1007/BF02427280

[29] Vilsbøll T, Holst JJ. Incretins, insulin secretion and Type 2 diabetes mellitus. Diabetologia. 2004;**47**(3):357-366. DOI: 10.1007/s00125-004-1342-6

[30] Vaag AA, Holst JJ, Vølund A, Beck-Nielsen H. Gut incretin hormones in identical twins discordant for non-insulin-dependent diabetes mellitus (NIDDM)—Evidence for decreased glucagon-like peptide 1 secretion during oral glucose ingestion in NIDDM twins. European Journal of Endocrinology. 1996;**135**(4):425-432

[31] Toft-Nielsen M-B, Damholt MB, Madsbad S, Hilsted LM, Hughes TE, Michelsen BK, et al. Determinants of the impaired secretion of glucagon-like peptide-1 in type 2 diabetic patients. The Journal of Clinical Endocrinology and Metabolism. 2001;**86**(8):3717-3723. DOI: 10.1210/jc.86.8.3717

[32] Holst JJ, Gromada J. Role of incretin hormones in the regulation of insulin secretion in diabetic and nondiabetic humans. American Journal of Physiology. Endocrinology and Metabolism. 2004;**287**(2):E199-E206. DOI: 10.1152/ajpendo.00545.2003

[33] Cassar S, Teede HJ, Harrison CL, Joham AE, Moran LJ, Stepto NK. Biomarkers and insulin sensitivity in women with Polycystic Ovary Syndrome: Characteristics and predictive capacity. Clinical Endocrinology (Oxford). 2015;**83**(1):50-58. DOI: 10.1111/cen.12619

[34] Gama R, Norris F, Wright J, Morgan L, Hampton S, Watkins K, et al. The entero-insular axis in polycystic ovarian syndrome. Annals of Clinical Biochemistry. 1996;**33**(3):190-195

[35] Svendsen PF, Nilas L, Madsbad S, Holst JJ. Incretin hormone secretion in women with polycystic ovary syndrome: Roles of obesity, insulin sensitivity, and treatment with metformin. Metabolism. 2009;**58**(5):586-593. DOI: 10.1016/j.metabol.2008.11.009

[36] Lin T, Li S, Xu H, Zhou H, Feng R, Liu W, et al. Gastrointestinal hormone secretion in women with polycystic ovary syndrome: An observational study. Human Reproduction (Oxford, England). 2015;**30**(11):2639-2644. DOI: 10.1093/humrep/dev231

[37] Aydin K, Arusoglu G, Koksal G, Cinar N, Yazgan Aksoy D, Yildiz BO. Fasting and postprandial glucagon like peptide 1 and oral contraception in polycystic ovary syndrome. Clinical Endocrinology (Oxford). 2014;**81**(4):588-592. DOI: 10.1111/cen.12468

[38] Chang CL, Huang SY, Soong YK, Cheng PJ, Wang C-J, Liang IT. Circulating irisin and glucose-dependent insulinotropic peptide are associated with the development of polycystic ovary syndrome. The Journal of Clinical Endocrinology and Metabolism. 2014;**99**(12):E2539-E2548. DOI: 10.1210/jc.2014-1180

[39] Thomson RL, Buckley JD, Noakes M, Clifton PM, Norman RJ, Brinkworth GD. The effect of a hypocaloric diet with and without exercise training on body composition, cardiometabolic risk profile, and reproductive function in overweight and obese women with polycystic ovary syndrome. The Journal of Clinical Endocrinology and Metabolism. 2008;**93**(9):3373-3380. DOI: 10.1210/jc.2008-0751

[40] Moran LJ, Hutchison SK, Norman RJ, Teede HJ. Lifestyle changes in women with polycystic ovary syndrome. Cochrane Database of Systematic Reviews. 2011;(7):CD007506. DOI: 10.1002/14651858.CD007506.pub3

[41] Haqq L, McFarlane J, Dieberg G, Smart N. Effect of lifestyle intervention on the reproductive endocrine profile in women with polycystic ovarian syndrome: A systematic review and meta-analysis. Endocrine Connections. 2014;**3**(1):36-46. DOI: 10.1530/EC-14-0010

[42] National Institute for Health and Clinical Excellence Obesity. Guidance on the Prevention, Identification, Assessment and Management of Overweight and Obesity in Adults and Children. NICE Clin Guidel 2006 [Internet] Available from: https://www.nice.org.uk/guidance/cg43 [Accessed: July 30, 2017]

[43] Clark AM, Ledger W, Galletly C, Tomlinson L, Blaney F, Wang X, et al. Weight loss results in significant improvement in pregnancy and ovulation rates in anovulatory obese women. Human Reproduction (Oxford, England). 1995;**10**(10):2705-2712

[44] Clark AM, Thornley B, Tomlinson L, Galletley C, Norman RJ. Weight loss in obese infertile women results in improvement in reproductive outcome for all forms of fertility treatment. Human Reproduction (Oxford, England). 1998;**13**(6):1502-1505. DOI: 10.1093/humrep/13.6.1502

[45] Huber-Buchholz MM, Carey DG, Norman RJ. Restoration of reproductive potential by lifestyle modification in obese polycystic ovary syndrome: Role of insulin sensitivity and luteinizing hormone. The Journal of Clinical Endocrinology and Metabolism. 1999;**84**(4):1470-1474. DOI: 10.1210/jcem.84.4.5596

[46] Marsh KA, Steinbeck KS, Atkinson FS, Petocz P, Brand-Miller JC. Effect of a low glycemic index compared with a conventional healthy diet on polycystic ovary syndrome. The American Journal of Clinical Nutrition. 2010;**92**(1):83-92. DOI: 10.3945/ajcn.2010.29261

[47] Kiddy DS, Hamilton-Fairley D, Bush A, Short F, Anyaoku V, Reed MJ, et al. Improvement in endocrine and ovarian function during dietary treatment of obese women with polycystic ovary syndrome. Clinical Endocrinology (Oxford). 1992;**36**(1):105-111. DOI: 10.1111/j.1365-2265.1992.tb02909.x

[48] Gambineri A, Pagotto U, Tschöp M, Vicennati V, Manicardi E, Carcello A, et al. Antiandrogen treatment increases circulating ghrelin levels in obese women with polycystic ovary syndrome. Journal of Endocrinological Investigation. 2003;**26**(7):629-634

[49] Nieuwenhuis-Ruifrok AE, Kuchenbecker WKH, Hoek A, Middleton P, Norman RJ. Insulin sensitizing drugs for weight loss in women of reproductive age who are overweight or obese: Systematic review and meta-analysis. Human Reproduction Update. 2009;**15**(1):57-68. DOI: 10.1093/humupd/dmn043

[50] Padwal R, Li SK, Lau DCW. Long-term pharmacotherapy for overweight and obesity: A systematic review and meta-analysis of randomized controlled trials. International Journal of Obesity and Related Metabolic Disorders: Journal of the International Association for the Study of Obesity. 2003;**27**(12):1437-1446. DOI: 10.1038/sj.ijo.0802475

[51] Lamos EM, Malek R, Davis SN. GLP-1 receptor agonists in the treatment of polycystic ovary syndrome. Expert Review of Clinical Pharmacology. 2017;**10**(4):401-408. DOI: 10.1080/17512433.2017.1292125

[52] Niafar M, Pourafkari L, Porhomayon J, Nader N. A systematic review of GLP-1 agonists on the metabolic syndrome in women with polycystic ovaries. Archives of Gynecology and Obstetrics. 2016;**293**(3):509-515. DOI: 10.1007/s00404-015-3976-7

[53] Jensterle Sever M, Kocjan T, Pfeifer M, Kravos NA, Janez A. Short-term combined treatment with liraglutide and metformin leads to significant weight loss in obese women with polycystic ovary syndrome and previous poor response to metformin. European Journal of Endocrinology. 2014;**170**(3):451-459. DOI: 10.1530/EJE-13-0797

[54] Jensterle M, Kravos NA, Pfeifer M, Kocjan T, Janez A. A 12-week treatment with the long-acting glucagon-like peptide 1 receptor agonist liraglutide leads to significant weight loss in a subset of obese women with newly diagnosed polycystic ovary syndrome. Hormones (Athens, Greece). 2015;**14**(1):81-90

[55] Rasmussen CB, Lindenberg S. The effect of liraglutide on weight loss in women with polycystic ovary syndrome: An observational study. Frontiers in Endocrinology. 2014;**5**:140. DOI: 10.3389/fendo.2014.00140

[56] Jensterle M, Kocjan T, Kravos NA, Pfeifer M, Janez A. Short-term intervention with liraglutide improved eating behavior in obese women with polycystic ovary syndrome. Endocrine Research. 2015;**40**(3):133-138. DOI: 10.3109/07435800.2014.966385

[57] Jensterle M, Goricar K, Janez A. Metformin as an initial adjunct to low-dose liraglutide enhances the weight-decreasing potential of liraglutide in obese polycystic ovary syndrome: Randomized control study. Experimental and Therapeutic Medicine. 2016;**11**:1194-1200. DOI: 10.3892/etm.2016.3081

[58] Kahal H, Aburima A, Ungvari T, Rigby AS, Coady AM, Vince RV, et al. The effects of treatment with liraglutide on atherothrombotic risk in obese young women with polycystic ovary syndrome and controls. BMC Endocrine Disorders. 2015;**15**:14. DOI: 10.1186/s12902-015-0005-6

[59] Elkind-Hirsch K, Marrioneaux O, Bhushan M, Vernor D, Bhushan R. Comparison of single and combined treatment with exenatide and metformin on menstrual cyclicity in overweight women with polycystic ovary syndrome. The Journal of Clinical Endocrinology and Metabolism. 2008;**93**(7):2670-2678. DOI: 10.1210/jc.2008-0115

[60] Jensterle M, Salamun V, Kocjan T, Vrtacnik Bokal E, Janez A. Short term monotherapy with GLP-1 receptor agonist liraglutide or PDE 4 inhibitor roflumilast is superior to metformin in weight loss in obese PCOS women: A pilot randomized study. Journal of Ovarian Research. 2015;**8**:32. DOI: 10.1186/s13048-015-0161-3

[61] Nylander M, Frøssing S, Clausen HV, Kistorp C, Faber J, Skouby SO. Effects of liraglutide on ovarian dysfunction in polycystic ovary syndrome: A randomized clinical trial. Reproductive Biomedicine Online. 2017;**35**(1):121-127. DOI: 10.1016/j.rbmo.2017.03.023

[62] Astrup A, Rössner S, Van Gaal L, Rissanen A, Niskanen L, Al Hakim M, et al. Effects of liraglutide in the treatment of obesity: A randomised, double-blind, placebo-controlled study. Lancet (London, England). 2009;**374**(9701):1606-1616. DOI: 10.1016/S0140-6736(09)61375-1

[63] Davies MJ, Bergenstal R, Bode B, Kushner RF, Lewin A, Skjøth TV, et al. Efficacy of liraglutide for weight loss among patients with type 2 diabetes: The SCALE diabetes randomized clinical trial. Journal of the American Medical Association. 2015;**314**(7):687-699. DOI: 10.1001/jama.2015.9676

[64] Vilsbøll T, Christensen M, Junker AE, Knop FK, Gluud LL. Effects of glucagon-like peptide-1 receptor agonists on weight loss: Systematic review and meta-analyses of randomised controlled trials. British Medical Journal. 2012;**344**:d7771. DOI: 10.1136/bmj.d7771

[65] Wilding JPH, Overgaard RV, Jacobsen LV, Jensen CB, le Roux CW. Exposure-response analyses of liraglutide 3.0 mg for weight management. Diabetes, Obesity & Metabolism. 2016;**18**(5):491-499. DOI: 10.1111/dom.12639

[66] Pi-Sunyer X, Astrup A, Fujioka K, Greenway F, Halpern A, Krempf M, et al. A randomized, controlled trial of 3.0 mg of liraglutide in weight management. The New England Journal of Medicine. 2015;**373**(1):11-22. DOI: 10.1056/NEJMoa1411892

[67] Wadden TA, Hollander P, Klein S, Niswender K, Woo V, Hale PM, et al. Weight maintenance and additional weight loss with liraglutide after low-calorie-diet-induced weight loss: The SCALE Maintenance randomized study. International Journal of Obesity (2005). 2013;**37**(11):1443-1451. DOI: 10.1038/ijo.2013.120

[68] Collier A, Blackman A, Foster G, Zammit G, Rosenberg R, Wadden T, et al. S28 liraglutide 3.0 mg reduces severity of obstructive sleep apnoea and body weight in obese individuals with moderate or severe disease: Scale sleep apnoea trial. Thorax. 2014;**69**(Suppl 2):A16-A17. DOI: 10.1136/thoraxjnl-2014-206260.34

[69] Skibicka KP. The central GLP-1: Implications for food and drug reward. Frontiers in Neuroscience. 2013;**7**:181. DOI: 10.3389/fnins.2013.00181

[70] Keskitalo K, Tuorila H, Spector TD, Cherkas LF, Knaapila A, Kaprio J, et al. The Three-Factor Eating Questionnaire, body mass index, and responses to sweet and salty fatty foods: A twin study of genetic and environmental associations. The American Journal of Clinical Nutrition. 2008;**88**(2):263-271

[71] Inoue K, Maeda N, Kashine S, Fujishima Y, Kozawa J, Hiuge-Shimizu A, et al. Short-term effects of liraglutide on visceral fat adiposity, appetite, and food preference: A pilot study of obese Japanese patients with type 2 diabetes. Cardiovascular Diabetology. 2011;**10**:109. DOI: 10.1186/1475-2840-10-109

[72] Maida A, Lamont BJ, Cao X, Drucker DJ. Metformin regulates the incretin receptor axis via a pathway dependent on peroxisome proliferator-activated receptor-α in mice. Diabetologia. 2011;**54**(2):339-349. DOI: 10.1007/s00125-010-1937-z

[73] Mannucci E, Ognibene A, Cremasco F, Bardini G, Mencucci A, Pierazzuoli E, et al. Effect of metformin on glucagon-like peptide 1 (GLP-1) and leptin levels in obese nondiabetic subjects. Diabetes Care. 2001;**24**(3):489-494. DOI: 10.2337/diacare.24.3.489

[74] Mannucci E, Tesi F, Bardini G, Ognibene A, Petracca MG, Ciani S, et al. Effects of metformin on glucagon-like peptide-1 levels in obese patients with and without Type 2 diabetes. Diabetes, Nutrition & Metabolism. 2004;**17**(6):336-342

[75] Yasuda N, Inoue T, Nagakura T, Yamazaki K, Kira K, Saeki T, et al. Enhanced secretion of glucagon-like peptide 1 by biguanide compounds. Biochemical and Biophysical Research Communications. 2002;**298**(5):779-784. DOI: 10.1016/S0006-291X(02)02565-2

[76] D'Alessio DA. What if gut hormones aren't really hormones: DPP-4 inhibition and local action of GLP-1 in the gastrointestinal tract. Endocrinology. 2011;**152**(8):2925-2926. DOI: 10.1210/en.2011-1385

[77] Jensterle M, Pirš B, Goričar K, Dolžan V, Janež A. Genetic variability in GLP-1 receptor is associated with inter-individual differences in weight lowering potential of liraglutide in obese women with PCOS: A pilot study. European Journal of Clinical Pharmacology. 2015;**71**:817-824. DOI: 10.1007/s00228-015-1868-1

[78] Kahal H, Abouda G, Rigby AS, Coady AM, Kilpatrick ES, Atkin SL. Glucagon-like peptide-1 analogue, liraglutide, improves liver fibrosis markers in obese women with polycystic ovary syndrome and nonalcoholic fatty liver disease. Clinical Endocrinology (Oxford). 2014;**81**(4):523-528. DOI: 10.1111/cen.12369

[79] Jensterle-Sever M, Šalamun V, Vrtačnik-Bokal E, Janež A. Short-term intervention with liraglutide and metformin increased fertility potential in a subset of obese women with PCOS proceeding in vitro fertilization. Endocrine Reviews. 2017;**38**(3 Suppl):SAT 095 DOI: 10.1186/s12902-017-0155-9. ISSN: 1945-7189

[80] Shimizu I, Hirota M, Ohboshi C, Shima K. Identification and localization of glucagon-like peptide-1 and its receptor in rat brain. Endocrinology. 1987;**121**(3):1076-1082. DOI: 10.1210/endo-121-3-1076

[81] Fabbri LM, Calverley PMA, Izquierdo-Alonso JL, Bundschuh DS, Brose M, Martinez FJ, et al. Roflumilast in moderate-to-severe chronic obstructive pulmonary disease treated with long-acting bronchodilators: Two randomised clinical trials. Lancet (London, England). 2009;**374**(9691):695-703. DOI: 10.1016/S0140-6736(09)61252-6

[82] Wouters EFM, Bredenbröker D, Teichmann P, Brose M, Rabe KF, Fabbri LM, et al. Effect of the phosphodiesterase 4 inhibitor roflumilast on glucose metabolism in patients with treatment-naive, newly diagnosed type 2 diabetes mellitus. The Journal of Clinical Endocrinology and Metabolism. 2012;**97**(9):E1720-E1725. DOI: doi.org/10.1210/jc.2011-2886

[83] Jensterle M, Kocjan T, Janez A. Phosphodiesterase 4 inhibition as a potential new therapeutic target in obese women with polycystic ovary syndrome. The Journal of Clinical Endocrinology and Metabolism. 2014;**99**(8):E1476-E1481. DOI: 10.1210/jc.2014-1430

[84] Vollert S, Kaessner N, Heuser A, Hanauer G, Dieckmann A, Knaack D, et al. The glucose-lowering effects of the PDE4 inhibitors roflumilast and roflumilast-N-oxide in db/db mice. Diabetologia. 2012;**55**(10):2779-2788. DOI: 10.1007/s00125-012-2632-z

[85] Amori RE, Lau J, Pittas AG. Efficacy and safety of incretin therapy in type 2 diabetes: Systematic review and meta-analysis. Journal of the American Medical Association. 2007;**298**(2):194-206. DOI: 10.1001/jama.298.2.194

[86] Khoo J, Rayner CK, Jones KL, Horowitz M. Incretin-based therapies: New treatments for type 2 diabetes in the new millennium. Therapeutics and Clinical Risk Management. 2009;**5**(3):683-698. DOI: 10.2147/TCRM.S4975

[87] Holst JJ, Deacon CF. Is there a place for incretin therapies in obesity and prediabetes? Trends in Endocrinology and Metabolism: TEM. 2013;**24**(3):145-152. DOI: 10.1016/j.tem.2013.01.004

[88] Phung OJ, Scholle JM, Talwar M, Coleman CI. Effect of noninsulin antidiabetic drugs added to metformin therapy on glycemic control, weight gain, and hypoglycemia in type 2 diabetes. Journal of the American Medical Association. 2010;**303**(14):1410-1418. DOI: 10.1001/jama.2010.405

[89] Aroda VR, Henry RR, Han J, Huang W, DeYoung MB, Darsow T, et al. Efficacy of GLP-1 receptor agonists and DPP-4 inhibitors: Meta-analysis and systematic review. Clinical Therapeutics. 2012;**34**(6):1247-1258.e22. DOI: 10.1016/j.clinthera.2012.04.013

[90] Intensive blood-glucose control with sulphonylureas or insulin compared with conventional treatment and risk of complications in patients with type 2 diabetes (UKPDS 33). UK Prospective Diabetes Study (UKPDS) Group. Lancet (London, England). 1998;**352**(9131):837-853. DOI: 10.1016/S0140-6736(98)07019-6

[91] Aulinger BA, Bedorf A, Kutscherauer G, de Heer J, Holst JJ, Göke B, et al. Defining the role of GLP-1 in the enteroinsulinar axis in type 2 diabetes using DPP-4 inhibition and GLP-1 receptor blockade. Diabetes. 2014;**63**(3):1079-1092. DOI: 10.2337/db13-1455

[92] Jensterle M, Goricar K, Janez A. Add on DPP-4 inhibitor alogliptin alone or in combination with pioglitazone improved β-cell function and insulin sensitivity in metformin treated PCOS. Endocrine Research. 2017;1-8. DOI: 10.1080/07435800.2017.1294602

[93] Ferjan S, Janež A, Jensterle M. Dipeptidyl peptidase-4 (DPP-4) inhibitor sitagliptin improved beta cell function and prevented a conversion rate to IGT and DM2 in metformin intolerant PCOS with high metabolic risk. Diabetes. 2017;**66**(Suppl. 1):A563

[94] Elkind-Hirsch KE, Paterson MS, Seidemann EL, Gutowski HC. Short-term therapy with combination dipeptidyl peptidase-4 inhibitor saxagliptin/metformin extended release (XR) is superior to saxagliptin or metformin XR monotherapy in prediabetic women with polycystic ovary syndrome: A single-blind, randomized, pilot study. Fertility and Sterility. 2017;**107**(1):253-260.e1. DOI: 10.1016/j.fertnstert.2016.09.023

[95] Jensterle Sever M, Ferjan S, Janež A. DPP4 inhibitor sitagliptin in combination with metformin prevent weight regain in obese women with PCOS previously treated with liraglutide. Endocrine Reviews. 2017;**38**(3 Suppl): OR 28-2. ISSN: 1945-7189 Available from: http://www.endocrine.org/meetings/endo-annual-meetings/abstract-details?ID=30608

[96] Bariatric Surgery Guidelines and Recommendations [Internet]. American Society for Metabolic and Bariatric Surgery. Available from: https://asmbs.org/resources/bariatric-surgery-guidelines-and-recommendations [Accessed: Jul 29, 2017]

[97] Morínigo R, Moizé V, Musri M, Lacy AM, Navarro S, Marín JL, et al. Glucagon-like peptide-1, peptide YY, hunger, and satiety after gastric bypass surgery in morbidly obese subjects. The Journal of Clinical Endocrinology and Metabolism. 2006;**91**(5):1735-1740. DOI: 10.1210/jc.2005-0904

[98] Evans S, Pamuklar Z, Rosko J, Mahaney P, Jiang N, Park C, et al. Gastric bypass surgery restores meal stimulation of the anorexigenic gut hormones glucagon-like peptide-1 and peptide YY independently of caloric restriction. Surgical Endoscopy. 2012;**26**(4):1086-1094

[99] Korner J, Bessler M, Cirilo LJ, Conwell IM, Daud A, Restuccia NL, et al. Effects of Roux-en-Y gastric bypass surgery on fasting and postprandial concentrations of plasma ghrelin, peptide YY, and insulin. The Journal of Clinical Endocrinology and Metabolism. 2005;**90**(1):359-365. DOI: 10.1210/jc.2004-1076

[100] Korner J, Bessler M, Inabnet W, Taveras C, Holst JJ. Exaggerated GLP-1 and blunted GIP secretion are associated with Roux-en-Y gastric bypass but not adjustable gastric banding. Surgery for Obesity and Related Diseases: Official Journal of the American Society for Bariatric Surgery. 2007;**3**(6):597-601

[101] Eid GM, Cottam DR, Velcu LM, Mattar SG, Korytkowski MT, Gosman G, et al. Effective treatment of polycystic ovarian syndrome with Roux-en-Y gastric bypass. Surgery for Obesity and Related Diseases. 2005;**1**(2):77-80. DOI: 10.1016/j.soard.2005.02.008

[102] Jamal M, Gunay Y, Capper A, Eid A, Heitshusen D, Samuel I. Roux-en-Y gastric bypass ameliorates polycystic ovary syndrome and dramatically improves conception rates:

A 9-year analysis. Surgery for Obesity and Related Diseases. 2012;**8**(4):440-444. DOI: 10.1016/j.soard.2011.09.022

[103] Stroh C, Hohmann U, Lehnert H, Manger T. PCO syndrome—Is it an indication for bariatric surgery? Zentralblatt fur Chirurgie. 2008;**133**(6):608-610. DOI: 10.1055/s-2008-1076869

[104] George K, Azeez H. Resolution of gynaecological issues after bariatric surgery—A retrospective analysis. Obesity Surgery. 2013;**23**(8):1043. DOI: 10.1007/s11695-013-0986-z

Chapter 6

Ovulation Induction in Women with Polycystic Ovary Syndrome: What is the Optimal Option?

Vaduneme K. Oriji and Kennedy Nyengidiki

Additional information is available at the end of the chapter

http://dx.doi.org/10.5772/intechopen.70812

Abstract

Infertility is a distressing medical and psychosocial problem afflicting about a quarter of all couples wanting to reproduce their offspring. Majority of the anovulatory problem in the female, as a cause of infertility, is due to polycystic ovary syndrome (PCOS). This condition is a complex interplay of factors, which affect women even beyond their fertility. It has been found to increase the risk of other adverse conditions such as the metabolic syndrome, cardiovascular diseases, type II diabetes mellitus, and endometrial cancer as well as infertility. Different groups have made diagnosis of PCOS with various diagnostic criteria. The Rotterdam criteria used in the diagnosis of PCOS mainly emphasize the reproductive malfunctions of this complex disease. The treatment of anovulatory infertility in PCOS is as enigmatic as the disease itself. Various methods have been deployed to treat the anovulation with variable success. Clomiphene citrate is a traditional first-line drug in treating anovulation in women with PCOS. Weight reduction, letrozole, metformin, follicle-stimulating hormone (FSH) and ovarian drilling are some of the other ways in which anovulation has been treated in these women. What method is more likely to succeed in treating the infertility from anovulation in PCOS and in what circumstance are the subject matters of this discussion.

Keywords: polycystic ovary syndrome, ovulation induction in PCOS, anovulatory infertility, clomiphene citrate, letrozole

1. Introduction

Polycystic ovarian syndrome (PCOS) is a group of heterogeneous endocrine disease affecting women characterized by irregular menses, hyperandrogenism, and polycystic ovaries. The diagnoses of polycystic ovarian syndrome are frequently made for the first time in the infertility clinic during evaluations for infertility. Infertility is the main clinical manifestation of ovulatory dysfunction in patients with PCOS. The prevalence is between 8.5 and 20% depending on the criteria used for the identification of the condition [1, 2].

Anovulation is a cause of infertility in up to a quarter of all cases of infertility. Normogonadotropic anovulation classified as World Health Organization (WHO) group II is the most common category of anovulatory infertility. PCOS is the most common in this group and notably the commonest endocrine disorder and cause of anovulation [1–3]. Insulin resistance is implicated in the ovulatory dysfunction in PCOS by disrupting the hypothalamo-pituitary-ovarian axis. Insulin resistance also leads to other comorbidities such as metabolic syndrome, hypertension, dyslipidemia, glucose intolerance, and diabetes mellitus as well as mental disorders such as depression, anxiety, bipolar disorders and binge eating [1, 4]. Women with PCOS present to the fertility clinic with chronic oligo/anovulation and hyperandrogenism, with attendant negative effects on their fertility. The desire to reproduce is very intense in many communities where there is high premium placed on reproduction as a means of survival. So, these women having learnt the diagnosis of their conditions are very expectant that their conditions will soon be reversed following treatment such that they could ovulate, become pregnant, and successfully have children. Many a times, the drug to bring about the reversal of anovulation refuses to work due to innate characteristics within the woman, the drug, or even the environment. This challenge has led to the development and use of several different pharmacologic agents used singularly and in combination to deal with the challenge of anovulation. Other physical methods and herbal preparations have also been deployed to varying degree of success to combat anovulation in women with PCOS.

Central to the management of women with infertility from PCOS is the induction of ovulation. The treatment options for infertility in women with PCOS include clomiphene citrate, gonadotropins, laparoscopic ovarian drilling (LOD), and assisted reproductive technology [1, 5]. Common to all methods is the induction of ovulation. Letrozole and metformin also play important roles in ovulation induction as has been now well demonstrated. The use of these pharmacologic agents has been shown to be superior to placebo or no treatment in terms of pregnancy or ovulation [6].

2. Weight reduction and ovulation induction

Scientific studies have not confirmed that women could regain spontaneous ovulation with voluntary weight loss and other life style modifications as systematic reviews did not identify studies that confirm that ovulation and other clinical reproductive outcomes improved with weight loss in women with PCOS but the studies identified increased total testosterone, androgen index, hirsute, fasting blood glucose, fasting insulin, and worsened lipid profile in the obese women compared with normal weight women with PCOS [7–9]. Obesity is linked to anolution and pregnancy loss as well as poor response with ovulation induction methods such as clomiphene citrate, gonadotropins, letrozole, and ovarian drilling [10–15]. This is important as previous authors have surmised that since obesity is found in some women with PCOS and worsens insulin resistance, that weight loss would improve ovulation and other reproductive outcomes [4, 16–19].

The American societies studying PCOS indicate that weight loss is a primary therapy in PCOS. That weight loss as little as 5–10% of body weight can regularize menses and improve response to ovulation induction and fertility medications [9, 12].

In many countries, lifestyle intervention is recommended as this has led to higher spontaneous ovulation rates and natural conception rates [20, 21].

Weight reduction through dietary modification and exercise is recommended for overweight PCOS patient [22]. Some studies show that over 10% of women with PCOS will regain spontaneous ovulation when placed on low calorie, low-fat diet, and exercise or with surgery. The aim of dietary restriction and exercise is toward losing about 5–10% of their body weight. This form of treatment alone or in combination with pharmacologic agents would reduce insulin resistance and is advocated for overweight to obese women of BMI > 24 [22]. The drawbacks of this method of treatment are that such women lack the motivation to remain on diet and exercise, and may not be able to achieve the desired weight loss to trigger spontaneous ovulation, and most times pharmacologic agents are added to assist ovulation. The duration it takes to achieve the desired body weight to bring about ovulation is not defined, but differs among patients. Other drawbacks are that it may not treat anovulation in normal-weight women even though they also have insulin resistance as well. The advantage is that it is cost-effective and will not produce any form of drug reactions. It will also reduce the high level of luteinizing hormone and reduce early pregnancy loss. A combination of lifestyle modification with weight loss before pharmacologic ovulation-inducing agents improved ovulation and live birth in women with PCOS in a USA study [23] and in addition, required lower doses of pharmacologic agent for ovulation induction.

3. Pharmacologic agents and ovulation induction

3.1. Use of pharmacologic agents in induction of ovulation

Several pharmacologic agents have been used to induce ovulation in these patients. They have achieved varied success with attendant setbacks from these drugs especially in achieving pregnancy and with adverse pregnancy outcomes. These drugs include clomiphene citrate, metformin, letrozole, gonadotropins, inositol, and tamoxifen.

3.1.1. Clomiphene citrate

Clomiphene citrate is traditionally the first-line drug used to induce ovulation in women with anovulation due to PCOS [2]. This drug has both estrogenic agonist and antagonist effects. It produces its effect principally by blocking the estrogen receptors in the hypothalamus to increase the endogenous follicle-stimulating hormone (FSH) to bring about folliculogenesis and ovulation. Clomiphene citrate when compared to other pharmacologic agents used for induction have been found to be inferior to drugs like letrozole, or a combination of clomiphene citrate and metformin with respect to ovulation, pregnancy, or live birth [6]. Clomiphene citrate in combination with metformin showed a higher pregnancy rate than clomiphene citrate alone or metformin alone. The odds ratio for pregnancy when clomiphene citrate in combination with metformin is compared to clomiphene citrate alone is 1.8 (1.35–2.42) indicating that clomiphene citrate in combination with metformin is a better treatment and offers 1.8 times the chance of pregnancy compared to the clomiphene citrate alone.

A small group patients do not ovulate at a maximum dose of 150 mg of clomiphene citrate for 5 days; they are taken to be clomiphene-resistant and anyone unable to achieve pregnancy for a period of 6 months on clomiphene citrate is termed to have clomiphene failure. Those resistant to clomiphene citrate will require other forms of ovulation induction, which may include a combination of the clomiphene citrate and metformin, other pharmacologic therapy or ovarian drilling to produce ovulation in this subset of women. Other disadvantages of clomiphene citrate are its antagonist effect on the estrogen receptors within the endometrium, which is thought to reduce the pregnancy rates in women treated with clomiphene citrate. The rates of multiple pregnancies with clomiphene citrate are below 10% and the risk of ovarian hyperstimulation is rare when compared to follicle stimulating hormone with higher chances of both multiple pregnancy and ovarian hyperstimulation syndrome [23]. The prolonged use of clomiphene may increase the risk development of uterine fibroid or endometrial cancer.

3.1.2. Letrozole

Letrozole is a third-generation aromatase inhibitor. In inducing ovulation, the drug acts primarily in the ovary where it antagonizes the effect of the enzyme 5α-reductase in the production of estrogen in the ovary. Its effect is to inhibit the conversion of testosterone and androstienedione to estradiol and estrone. It also blocks the conversion of androgen to estrogens in the peripheral fat cells and suppresses local estrogen production in the brain. The reduced levels of estrogen release the hypothalamus from the negative feedback effects of estrogen and cause increased production of FSH for folliculogenesis and ovulation.

Letrozole has been found to be superior to clomiphene citrate alone or even clomiphene citrate in combination with metformin. The systemic review and meta-analysis of the Rui Wang group showed that Letrozole produced a higher pregnancy and ovulation rates when compared with clomiphene citrate alone. The odds ratio for pregnancy or ovulation with letrozole compared with clomiphene citrate is 1.58 and 1.99, respectively. Similar outcome was also noted when compared to tamoxifen (another estrogen antagonist similar to clomiphene citrate).

Letrozole also led to higher live-birth rates when compared to clomiphene citrate alone. The chances of birth with letrozole are about 1.6 times higher than clomiphene. It also resulted in lower multiple pregnancy rates compared to the clomiphene citrate. In these regards, Letrozole is better than the clomiphene citrate used traditionally to induce ovulation in women with PCOS. However, the systematic review acceptably did not review the negative effects of these drugs. It also found that the risks of abortions are lower with letrozole group [6]. In patients with clomiphene citrate resistance, Letrozole in combination with metformin showed better efficacy than clomiphene-metformin combination in terms of ovulation rates, pregnancy rates, and live births rates. It also has less abortion rates in the meta-analysis of treatments of patients with clomiphene citrate-resistant PCOS [24].

Letrozole can be used as a first-line drug in the treatment of anovulation because of its higher ovulation, pregnancy and live birth rates, and lower multiple pregnancy rates. The main advantage of letrozole over clomiphene citrate or clomiphene citrate combination with metformin is the absence of anti-estrogenic effects at the level of the endometrium, which perhaps is responsible for its higher pregnancy and live birth rates [1]. Despite the promising results with letrozole, neither letrozole nor metformin is approved for the treatment of anovulation in many countries and it is outrightly prohibited in several other countries.

3.1.3. Metformin

Metformin is an oral hypoglycemic agent; a biguanide used for treatment of type 2 diabetes mellitus. It works as insulin sensitizer and reduces insulin resistance, which is a feature in PCOS. It improves ovulation and other reproductive functions. It assists in weight reduction and its effect is better in obese women with PCOS. Alone, metformin is a weak induction agent. However, it is very effective when used along with clomiphene citrate for the induction of ovulation in the patients with PCOS. When metformin is given in combination with clomiphene citrate, there were significantly higher pregnancy rates than metformin or clomiphene citrate alone. The chances of pregnancy increased over 1.7 times in those with the combination of clomiphene and metformin when compared to metformin alone. Letrozole and metformin are also superior to metformin or letrozole alone in inducing ovulation. However, metformin is also useful after ovarian drilling. It reduces insulin resistance and androgens levels, and increases ovulation and pregnancy rates in clomiphene citrate-resistant PCOS after laparoscopic ovarian drilling (LOD).

3.1.4. Gonadotropins

The gonadotropins have been used to bring about ovulation in several anovulatory conditions including PCOS. It acts directly on the primordial follicles replacing endogenous gonadotropins to bring about folliculogenesis and ovulation. All forms of gonadotropins ranging from the human menopausal gonadotropins (HMG) to the highly purified follicle stimulating hormone have been recognized to cause ovulation in women. The active agent is the follicle stimulating hormone. The major set back has been that it cannot be administered orally. When compared to other pharmacologic agents, the efficacy of the follicle-stimulating hormone in bringing about ovulation is the highest. It also has the highest live birth rates after letrozole in the network meta-analysis comparing the efficacy in the use of these agents [6]. In the patient with clomiphene resistance, FSH was superior to clomiphene-metformin combination in ovulation rates, pregnancy, and live birth rates as well [1]. The follicle-stimulating hormone led to a higher multiple pregnancy rates when compared to the other pharmacologic agents with a higher risk of ovarian hyperstimulation syndrome. These are the two most serious side effects of gonadotropins resulting from simultaneous growth of many follicles [6, 18, 25]. Gonadotropins could be the second-line drug for clomiphene-resistant PCOS patients [26, 27].

4. Surgery and ovulation induction

4.1. Use of ovarian drilling to induce ovulation

Laparoscopic ovarian drilling has been demonstrated to induce ovulation in women with PCOS. This method of ovulation induction is used for clomiphene-resistant and FSH-resistant PCOS.

The mechanism involved in the ovarian diathermy is that it leads to the correction of hypersecretion of LH brought about by modification of the ovarian pituitary feedback. The practice is to drill into both ovaries. However, unilateral drilling has been found to bring about ovulation in either ovaries as well [1, 15, 26]. A net meta-analysis comparing its use as an ovulation induction agent did not find it superior to placebo or no treatment. It had no significantly higher chance at pregnancy or higher pregnancy rates in women with PCOS [6]. In patients with clomiphene resistance where it is being advocated, LOD was found to reduce testosterone and Luteinising hormone levels and associated with more regular cycles, higher ovulation and pregnancy rates compared to metformin alone even though metformin results in more attenuation of luteinizing hormone [28]. Emerging evidence shows that unilateral ovarian drilling has similar effects as bilateral ovarian drilling in bringing about ovulation, pregnancy rates, and life birth rates. Reported pregnancy rates are lower than in treatment with HMG [24]. The seeming comparative advantage of LOD is in its one-off therapy, especially in patients with clomiphene citrate resistance, sustained reversal of the pathology, high ovulation and pregnancy rates, reduced risk of multiple pregnancy, and ovarian hyperstimulation syndrome as well as patient's acceptability [26]. LOD with elecrocautery was found to be superior in treating anovulation compared to laser drilling or use of gonadotropins in clomiphene-resistant PCOS patients. The major side effects of LOD are the fact that it is a theater procedure and requires anesthesia; it may reduce ovarian reserve and has been associated with peri-ovarian adhesions [29, 30]. When ranked according to efficacy of ovulation induction, the systemic review found out that the clomiphene citrate in combination with metformin was the most efficacious followed by follicle-stimulating hormone, letrozole, metformin, clomiphene, tamoxifen, laparoscopic ovarian drilling, and placebo or no treatment in that order. This when ranked in percentage efficacy of effectiveness showed 90, 82, 80, 50, 46, 27, 22 and 3%, respectively [6].

4.2. Use of bariatric surgery to induce ovulation

Bariatric surgery has been used for weight reduction among highly obese women who had bariatric surgery for just weight reduction. The bariatric surgery in obese PCOS patient also resulted in weight loss, spontaneous ovulation, and pregnancy.

5. Conclusion

However, when the ranking in terms of live birth rate was done, letrozole (81%) gave the best result, followed by follicle-stimulating hormone (74%), clomiphene-metformin (71%), tamoxifen (48%), clomiphene citrate (36%), metformin (30%), placebo or no treatment (10%).

Women with PCOS should undergo pre-conception counseling before any treatment for infertility. The importance of life-style modification, especially weight loss and exercise, should be emphasized and encouraged in overweight women, and smoking and alcohol consumption should be discouraged [24]. More randomized trial to determine the effect of weight loss to ovulation should be undertaken to elucidate clearly the place of weight loss as a means of ovulation of induction considering its affordability and acceptability as a means of treatment.

The controversy with the method of treating anovulatory infertility in women with PCOS will continue for some time. The systemic review found out that the clomiphene citrate in combination with metformin was the most efficacious followed by follicle-stimulating hormone, letrozole, metformin, clomiphene, tamoxifen, laparoscopic ovarian drilling, and placebo or no treatment in that order. However, when the ranking in terms of live birth rate was done, letrozole, follicle-stimulating hormone, clomiphene-metformin, tamoxifen, clomiphene citrate, metformin, placebo or no treatment was noted. It will therefore seem reasonable to include letrozole, clomiphene citrate and the combination of clomiphene citrate with metformin as possible first-line drugs in the treatment of anovulatory infertility in women with PCOS. While the gonadotropins is reserved as a second-line drug for these women, ovarian drilling is recommended after failure with the gonadotropins or whenever laparoscopy is indicated for any other reason in these women with failed clomiphene resistance. It will be advisable to refer patients that fail to achieve pregnancy using the methods above for assisted reproductive therapy for the treatment of their anovulatory infertility.

Author details

Vaduneme K. Oriji* and Kennedy Nyengidiki

*Address all correspondence to: vadoriji@yahoo.com

University of Port Harcourt and University of Port Harcourt Teaching Hospital, Port Harcourt, Nigeria

References

[1] Sirmans SM, Pate KA. Epidemiology, diagnosis, and management of polycystic ovary syndrome. Clinical Epidemiology. 2014;**6**:1-13. DOI: 10.2147/CLEP.S37559

[2] Broekmans FJ, Knauff EA, Valkenburg O, et al. PCOS a clomiphene citrate ording to the Rotterdam consensus criteria: Change in prevalence among WHO-II anovulation and association with metabolic factors. British Journal of Obstetrics and Gynaecology. 2006;**113**(10):1210-1217. DOI: 10.1111/j.1471-0528.2006.01008.x

[3] ESHRE Capri Workshop Group. Health and fertility in World Health Organization group 2 anovulatory women. Human Reproduction Update. 2012;**18**:586-599. DOI: 10.1093/humupd/dms019

[4] Goodman NF, Cobin RH, Futterweit W, Glueck JS, Legro RS, Carmine E, et al. American Association of Clinical Endocrinologists, American College of Endocrinology, and Androgen Excess and PCOS Society Disease State clinical review: Guide to the best practices in the evaluation and treatment of polycystic ovary syndrome – Part 1. Endocrine Practice. 2015;**21**(11):1291-1300. DOI: 10.4158/EP15748.DSC

[5] Guzick DS. Ovulation induction management of PCOS. Clinical Obstetrics and Gynecology. 2007;**50**(1):255-267. DOI: 10.1097/GRF.0b013e31802f361e

[6] Wang R, Kim BV, Wely MV, Johnson NP, Costello MF, Zhang H, Ng EHY. Treatment strategies for women with WHO group II anovulation: Systematic review and network meta-analysis. British Medical Journal. 2017;**356**:j136. DOI: https://doi.org/10.1136/bmj.j138

[7] Moran LJ, Hutchison SK, Norman RJ, Teede HJ. Lifestyle changes in women polycystic ovarian syndrome. Cochrane Database of Systematic Reviews. 2011 Feb 16;(2):CD007506. DOI: 10.1002/14651858

[8] Lim SS, Norman RJ, Davies MJ, et al. The effect of obesity on polycystic ovary syndrome: A systematic review and meta-analysis. Obesity Reviews. 2013;**14**(2):95-109. DOI: 10.1111/j.1467-789X.2012.01053.x

[9] Goodman NH, Cobin RH, Futterweit W, Gluec JS, Legro RS, Camina E. American Association of Clinical Endocrinologist, American College of Endocrinology and Androgen Excess and PCOS Society disease state clinical review: Guide to the best practices in the evaluation and treatment of polycystic ovarian syndrome – Part 2. Endocrine Practice. 2015;**21**(12):1415-1426

[10] Pasquali R, Pelusi C, Genghini S, Caciari M, Gambineri A. Obesity and reproductive disorders in women. Human Reproduction Update. 2003;**9**(4):359-372. DOI: org/10.1093/humupd/dmg024

[11] Mulders AG, Laven JS, Eijkemans MJ, Hughes EG, Fauser BC. Patient predictors for outcome of gonadotrophin ovulation induction in women with normogonadotrophic anovulatory infertility: A meta-analysis. Human Reproduction Update. 2003;**9**(5):429-449. DOI: doi.org/10.1093/humupd/dmg035

[12] Balen AH, Platteau P, Andersen AN, Devroey P, Sorensen P, Helmgaard L. The influence of body weight on response to ovulation induction with gonadotrophin in 335 women with World Health Organization group II anovulatory infertility. BJOG: An International Journal of Obstetrics and Gynaecology. 2006;**113**:1195-1202. DOI: 10.1111/j.1471-0528.2006.01034.x

[13] Froen JF, Arnestad M, Frey K, Vege A, Saugstad OD, Stray-Pedersen B. Risk factors for sudden intrauterine unexplained death: Epidemiologic characteristics of singleton cases in Oslo, Norway,1986–1995. American Journal of Obstetrics and Gynecology. 2001;**184**(4):694-702

[14] Imani B, Eijkemans MJ, te Velde ER, Habbema JD, Fauser BC. Predictors of patients remaining anovulatory during clomiphene citrate induction of ovulation in nomogonadotropic oligoamenorrheic infertility. The Journal of Clinical Endocrinology and Metabolism 1998;**83**(7):2361-2365. DOI: 10.1210/jcem.83.7.4919

[15] Gjonnaess H. Ovarian electrocautery in the treatment of women with polycystic ovary syndrome (PCOS). Factors affecting the results. Acta Obstetricia et Gynecologica Scandinavica. 1994;**73**(5):407-412

[16] Pasquali R, Gambeneri A, Pagotto U. The impact of obesity on reproduction in women with polycystic ovary syndrome. British Journal of Obstetrics and Gynaecology. 2006;**113**(10): 1148-1159. DOI: 10.1111/j.1471-0528.2006.00990.x

[17] Allahbadia GN, Merchant R. Polycystic ovary syndrome in the Indian Subcontinent. Seminars in Reproductive Medicine. 2008;**26**(1):22-34. DOI: 10.1055/s-2007-992921

[18] Yu Ng EH, Ho PC. Polycystic ovary syndrome in Asian women. Seminars in Reproductive Medicine. 2008;**26**(1):14-21. DOI: 10.1055/s-2007-992920 103.

[19] Homburg R. The management of infertility associated with polycystic ovary syndrome. Reproductive Biology and Endocrinology. 2003;**1**:109. DOI: 10.1186/1477-7827-1-109

[20] Legro RS, Dodson WC, Kris-Etherton PM, et al. Randomized controlled trial of preconception interventions in infertile women with polycystic ovary syndrome. The Journal of Clinical Endocrinology and Metabolism. 2015;**100**:4048-4058. DOI: 10.1210/jc.2015-2778

[21] Mutsaerts MA, van Oers AM, Groen H, et al. Randomized trial of a lifestyle program in obese infertile women. The New England Journal of Medicine. 2016;**374**:1942-1953. DOI: 10.1056/NEJMoa1505297.

[22] Badawy A, Elnashar A. Treatment options for polycystic ovary syndrome. International Journal of Women's Health. 2011;**3**:25. DOI: 10.2147/IJWH.S11304

[23] Legro RS, Dodson WC, Kunselman AR, et al. Benefit of delayed fertility therapy with preconception weight loss over immediate therapy in obese women with PCOS. The Journal of Clinical Endocrinology and Metabolism. 2016;**101**:2658-2666. DOI: 10.1210/jc.2016-1659

[24] Yiping Y, Fang L, Zhang R, He J, Xiong Y, Guo X, Qingyun D, et al. Comparative effectiveness of 9 ovulation-induction therapies in patients with clomiphene citrate-resistant polycystic ovary syndrome: A network meta-analysis. Scientific Reports. 2017; **7**:3812. DOI: 10.1038/s41598-017-03803-9

[25] Okohue J, Oriji VK, Ikimalo JI. Experience with bonano catheter in the management of ovarian hyperstimulation syndrome (OHSS) from IVF-ET treatment cycles. Nigerian Journal of Clinical Practice. 2017;**14**(4):428-431. DOI: 10.4103/1119-3077.212440

[26] Tehrani FR, Behboudi-Gandevani S. In: Contemporary Gynaecologic Practice. Darwish A, editor. Intech Publishers, Rijeka Croatia. 2015. DOI: org/10.5772/59591

[27] Thesoliniki ESHRE/ASRAM – Sponsored Consensus Workshop Group. Consensus on infertility treatment related to polycystic ovary syndrome. Fertility and Sterility. 2008;**89**(3): 505-522

[28] Hamed HO, Hasan AF, Ahmed OG, Ahmed MA. Metformin versus laparoscopic ovarian drilling in clomiphene- and insulin-resistant women with polycystic ovary syndrome. International Journal of Gynecology and Obsterics. 2010;**108**(2):143-147. DOI: 10.1016/j.ijgo.2009.08.033

[29] Oriji VK. Laparoscopic ovarian drilling versus medical treatment of in management of clomiphene citrate resistant polycystic ovary syndrome. World Journal of Laparoscopic Surgeries. 2010;**3**(2):99-102

[30] Saleh AM, Khalil HS. Review of nonsurgical and surgical treatment and the role of insulin-sensitizing agents in the management of infertile women with polycystic ovary syndrome. Acta Obstetricia et Gynecologica Scandinavica. 2004;**83**(7):614-621. DOI: 10.1111/j.0001-6349.2004.00481.x

Section 4

Complementary Therapies

Chapter 7

Complementary Therapy with Traditional Chinese Medicine for Polycystic Ovarian Syndrome

Yen-Nung Liao, Wen-Long Hu and Yu-Chiang Hung

Additional information is available at the end of the chapter

http://dx.doi.org/10.5772/intechopen.71654

Abstract

Polycystic ovarian syndrome (PCOS) is a common, heterogeneous, complex, endocrinopathic condition that causes menstrual dysfunction and infertility in women. Traditional Chinese medicine (TCM) has been widely used for PCOS in Far-East countries for thousands of years. There are significant advantages in treating PCOS with TCM. This chapter aims to investigate the current developments in TCM therapy for PCOS.

Keywords: complementary and alternative therapy, traditional Chinese medicine, polycystic ovarian syndrome, acupuncture, moxibustion

1. Introduction

1.1. Definition

Polycystic ovarian syndrome (PCOS) is characterized by endocrine and ovarian disorders that affect quality of life in women of reproductive age. In 1935, PCOS was first described by Stein and Leventhal with a description of seven women suffering from amenorrhea, hirsutism, and enlarged ovaries with multiple cysts [1, 2]. Some different criteria about the National Institute of Health (NIH), Rotterdam criteria, Androgen Excess Society and Polycystic Ovary Syndrome Society guidelines (AE-PCOS) are shown in **Table 1** [3–8].

1.2. Epidemiology

Globally, PCOS affects 5–20% of women of reproductive age [9]. One report summarized the incidence of PCOS as 6–13% in Hispanic women, 3–9% in African American women, and 2–9% in Asian women [10]. The prevalence of PCOS in different geographical regions ranges from

Title	NIH 1992	Rotterdam 2003	AE-PCOS 2006	NIH 2012 extension of Rotterdam 2003
Criteria	• Clinical or biochemical androgen excess • Rare ovulations	• Clinical or biochemical androgen excess • Oligo- or anovulation • Polycystic ovaries	• Clinical or biochemical androgen excess • Ovarian dysfunction and/or polycystic ovaries	• Clinical or biochemical androgen excess • Oligo- or anovulation • Polycystic ovaries
Restriction	Need both criteria	Need two of three criteria	Need both criteria	• Need two of three criteria • Specifically identifying the four sub-phenotype: A. Androgen Excess + Ovulatory Dyfunction + Polycystic Ovaries B. Androgen Excess + Ovulatory Dysfunction C. Androgen Excess + Polycystic Ovaries D. Ovulatory Dysfunction + Polycystic Ovarian Morphology
Exclusion	Exclusion of other androgen excess and other similar etiology			

Table 1. Diagnostic criteria for PCOS.

5 to 10% according to the NIH 1990 criteria, from 10 to 15% according to the AE-PCOS 2006 criteria, and from 6 to 21% when the Rotterdam criteria are applied [7]. East Asian subjects (Korean, Chinese, and Thai) appear to have a lower prevalence of PCOS (about 5%) compared to Caucasian women (11–20%) [11].

One systematic review and meta-analysis showed the incidence of PCOS phenotypes using the 2012 NIH criteria was 50% for phenotype A, 13% for phenotype B, 14% for phenotype C, and 17% for phenotype D [12].

1.3. Comorbidities

Patients with PCOS often have comorbidities such as obesity, insulin resistance/type II diabetes mellitus (Type II DM), dyslipidemia, hypertension/cardiovascular disease, infertility/subfertility, or cancer. One systematic review and meta-analysis demonstrated that women with PCOS had a pooled prevalence of 61% for overweight [body mass index (BMI) > 25], 49% for obesity (BMI > 30), and 54% for central obesity [13]. Insulin resistance (IR) is present in 50–80% of these women, which is associated with obesity [14, 15]. Both lean (30%) and obese women (70%) with PCOS show decreased insulin sensitivity [16].

Around 27% of premenopausal women with PCOS have type II DM [17]. Dyslipidemia may be up to 70% in women with PCOS [18, 19]. In a large study of European and American women with PCOS, the total cholesterol and low-density lipoprotein cholesterol (LDL-C) levels increased significantly, up to 29 and 16 mg/dl, respectively, in non-Hispanic white, obese women with PCOS compared to obese women without PCOS [19]. This study also noted that the total cholesterol and LDL-C levels were elevated significantly, up to 32 and 32 mg/dl, respectively, in nonobese women with PCOS compared to nonobese women without PCOS [19]. Another worldwide systematic review and meta-analysis demonstrated that triglycerides (TG) and LDL-C levels were 26 and 12 mg/dl higher, and high-density lipoprotein cholesterol (HDL-cholesterol) concentration was 6 mg/dl lower than that of controls [20].

One clinical study demonstrated that nearly 26% of women with PCOS have hypertension [21]. The metabolic imbalances in patients with PCOS cause chronic low-grade inflammation and cardiovascular disturbances, which increase the risk of cardiovascular disease [22]. One systematic review and meta-analysis showed a 2-fold increased risk of coronary heart disease (CHD) and stroke for women with PCOS compared to those without PCOS [23].

Women with PCOS account for around 80% of women with anovulatory infertility [24, 25]. A recently systematic review and meta-analysis showed that women of all ages with PCOS were at a significantly increased risk [odds ratio (OR) up to 2.79] for endometrial cancer [26]. Moreover, this study also revealed that when women over 54 years of age were excluded from the analysis, the risk for women with PCOS increased more (OR up to 4.05) for endometrial cancer and for ovarian cancer (OR up to 2.52), but stable for breast cancer [26].

2. Etiology

The etiology of PCOS is still not clear. A systematic review suggested that post-natal exposure to androgens results in reprogramming of the hypothalamic-pituitary-ovarian-axis [27]. Recently, some clinical studies have confirmed that human fetal androgen excess promotes PCOS development after birth by checking infant blood levels at term [28]. The circulating androgen levels of the human female fetus in the second trimester can increase into the male range and mid-gestational amniotic testosterone levels in female fetuses of PCOS mothers may be higher than those in normal mothers, which might influence fetal development [28]. Another review article mentioned that the fetal ovary is more likely to produce an excess of androgens in response to maternal human chorionic gonadotropin (hCG) in subjects genetically predisposed to PCOS [29]. Furthermore, some genetic variations are associated with PCOS. For example, DENND1A is found in the cytoplasm and nuclei of ovarian theca cells. Over expression of DENND1A variant 2 results in a PCOS-like phenotype, and knock-down of DENND1A variant 2 in PCOS theca cells reversed this phenotype [30]. In addition, a recent review showed that genome-wide association studies (GWAS) have identified some loci containing genes with clear roles in reproductive (LHCGR, FSHR, and FSHB) and metabolic (INSR and HMGA2) dysfunction in PCOS [31].

3. Diagnosis

There are several diagnostic criteria for PCOS such as NIH 1990/2012, ESHRE/ASRM 2003 (Rotterdam), or AE-PCOS 2006. Diagnosis of PCOS should take into consideration the history, clinical manifestations, ultrasound imaging results, and serum examination results.

3.1. History taking

Menstrual abnormality such as oligo-anovulation (OA) is usually noted [32]. According to the Rotterdam criteria, OA is defined as less than eight episodes of menses a year or cycle lengths of more than 35 days [5]. A stricter definition, such as less than eight menstruations and/or two cycles of less than 22 or more than 42 days per year, the prevalence of OA drops to 14% and OA becomes highly predictive of PCOS [33, 34]. Although 30% of women with PCOS will have normal menses [2, 35], 85–90% of women with OA have PCOS, while 30–40% of women with amenorrhea have PCOS [2, 36]. After the age of 40, women with PCOS often have more regular menstrual cycles while women over 30 who develop OA are less likely to have PCOS [32].

Weight gain and central obesity are common presentations in PCOS and usually come before the onset of anovulatory cycles [14]. In the United States, the prevalence of obesity in girls aged 12–19 years in 2007–2008 was 17%, compared with 50–80% among adolescent girls with PCOS [13, 37–40].

3.2. Clinical manifestations

Clinical manifestations are acne, hirsutism, and androgenic alopecia . Some patients appear with only one or two manifestations, while a few patients have all the three [2]. Sixty percent of patients with PCOS have hirsutism and 15–25% patients have acne [6].

3.3. Other diagnostic methods

The BMI, blood pressure, waist circumference (WC), and hip circumference should be measured at the initial visit. Fasting lipid profile, sugar and glycohemoglobin, or a 2-hour oral glucose tolerance test (OGTT) should be performed if PCOS is suspected at the initial visit. Trans-vaginal ultrasound is indicated rather than trans-abdominal ultrasound if the patient has one of either irregular menstruation or HA. The Rotterdam PCOM criteria, considered to have sufficient specificity and sensitivity to define PCOM, requires the presence of ≥12 follicles measuring 2–9 mm in diameter and/or increased ovarian volume (>10 cm^3) in a single ovary or both ovaries [32, 41–42]. In 2014, the AE-PCOS guidelines suggested using follicle number per ovary (FNPO) ≥25 for the definition of PCOM when using newer technology that allows maximal resolution of ovarian follicles (such as a transducer frequency of more than 8 MHz) [41, 43].

Serum hormone examination, such as serum androgens, should be performed on women with clinical appearance of PCOS. In addition, anti-Müllerian hormone (AMH) in women is generated by granulosa cells, and preantral and antral follicles, and its major function seems to be limited to inhibit the development of the initial stage of follicular maturation [44]. Serum

AMH in women with PCOS is higher than in healthy women, which probably reflects the number of small follicles observed on the ultrasounds of polycystic ovaries [45]. Studies have reported that 97% of women with AMH >10 ng/mL had PCOS and this correlated positively with LH, total testosterone, and DHEA [45, 46]. Besides, serum AMH revealed high predictive ability for the presence of OA or amenorrhea [45, 46]. Recently, serum AMH is proving to be a better tool to understand ovarian function and follicular count; however, the clinical use of serum assays for AMH still poses some technical problems [33, 44].

4. Conventional management and limitations

Management of PCOS is limited to improve clinical manifestations, since the real etiology of the disorder is unclear [47]. While multiple cardiovascular risk factors such as obesity, dyslipidemia, hypertension, and DM are prevalent in PCOS, current therapeutic management of PCOS usually focuses firstly on the treatment of metabolic disturbances (anovulation, menstrual irregularity, and hirsutism) and secondly on the control of reproductive hormones or insulin levels [48]. Lifestyle modifications including increased exercise, dietary changes, and weight loss are appropriate first-line interventions for many women with PCOS [49]. Diet therapy for patients with PCOS includes the design of low-calorie diets to achieve weight loss or preserve a healthy weight, restrict the intake of simple sugars, and increase the consumption of foods with a low glycemic index and refined carbohydrates, a decrease in the consumption of trans and saturated fatty acids, and awareness of possible deficiencies such as omega-3, vitamin D, and chromium [50]. One systematic review and meta-analysis demonstrated that moderate physical activity mostly 12 or 24 weeks would improve ovulation, decreased IR (9–30%), and weight loss (4.5–10%) [51]. The AE-PCOS guidelines suggested a target of caloric, diet, and body weight control in PCOS women with more restrictions if dyslipidemia occurred [52–54]. The detailed information is listed in **Table 2** [52–54].

Nutrition recommendations	Methods
Limitation of calories	Decrease current diet 500–1000 kcal/day
Reduction of fat	Decrease total fat (less than 30% total caloric intake) and saturated fat (less than 10% total caloric intake)
Favor foods intake	Increase fiber, vegetables, fruit, cereals, wholegrain breads, monounsaturated and polyunsaturated fat intake
Suggestions if dyslipidemia	**Expect reduction in LDL-C (%)**
Reduce body weight by 7–10%	5–8%
Decrease saturated fat to 7% total energy	8–10%
Decrease dietary cholesterol to <200 mg daily	3–5%
Decrease transfat to 1% total energy	2%
Increase 2 g of plant stanols daily	6–0%
Add 5–10 g viscous fiber daily	3–5%

Table 2. Nutritional recommendations for PCOS women from the AE-PCOS society.

Medical agents	Indication and effect	Limitations
Clomiphene citrate	*As an ovary-stimulating drug in subfertile /infertile women *Nonsteroidal synthetic hormone consisting of a racemic mixture of two stereoisomers (40% enclomiphene [EnC] and 60% zuclomiphene [ZuC]), with anti-estrogenic properties	*Possible fetal malformations, mainly neural tube defects and hypospadias *Increased risk of endometrial cancer, especially at doses greater than 2000 mg and high (more than 7) number of cycles
Metformin	*Usually used in young girls and adolescents with PCOS as first-line monotherapy or in combination with anti-androgen medications and OCPs *Improve hyperandrogenemia and symptoms of androgen excess *Recovery ovary function with normal menses *Assist in weight reduction *Reduce in metabolic parameters of insulin resistance	*Promoting ovulation is still controversial *Maybe increase IR after a 2-year period of intervention
Oral conceptions	*Contain estrogen (almost exclusively ethinylestradiol) and a progestin *Decrease androgens and block the effect of androgens by inhibiting of ovarian androgen production and by increasing SHBG *Advantageously combined with an anti-androgen to attain a better effect when treating hirsutism and alopecia	*Progestins, such as chlormadinone and drospirenone, may increase venous thrombosis events and may be contraindicated in severe obesity patients. *Little effect in blocking mild to moderate hirsutism or alopecia with OCPs only
Anti-androgens	*Competitive antagonism of the androgen receptor (spironolactone (SPA), cyproterone acetate, flutamide) or suppression of 5α-reductase (5αR, such as finasteride) to prevent the conversion of 5α-dihydrotestosterone into free testosterone *Suppress the effects of androgen in the hair follicle or in the pilosebaceous unit	*SPA may induce hyperkalemia, breast discomfort, dry skin, gastritis, headaches and dizziness *Intermenstrual spotting may occur if the women taking SPA as monotherapy *SPA has the potential for teratogenicity
Steroids	*Physiologic doses of prednisolone or dexamethasone can reduce androgen output directly	*Less effective for the treatment of hirsutism
Statins	*Lipid-lowering agents with multiple actions to improve dyslipidemia *Combined with an OCP can improve hirsutism	*Statins alone do not improve hirsutism, menstruation, or BMI

Table 3. Current medical agents and limitations for PCOS.

Unfortunately, lifestyle interventions are associated with low adherence and sustainability, and engagement, compliance, and sustainability remain challenging [55]. Medical treatment of PCOS is indicated if lifestyle modifications are a failure or unsuitable. Medical treatments include clomiphene citrate, metformin, oral contraceptives (OCPs), anti-androgen, steroids, and statins. One-year randomized clinical trial (RCT) showed that combined oral contraceptives plus spironolactone can decrease hirsutism score, androgens, and DHEA levels with fewer menstrual dysfunction [56]. Another randomized, controlled crossover study demonstrated that both metformin and myoinositol significantly reduced the insulin response to OGTT and improved insulin sensitivity [57]. Metformin could reduce body weight, improve menstrual pattern, and decrease LH, oestradiol levels, androgens, and AMH levels [57]. **Table 3** lists the medical treatment agents and limitations for PCOS [58–67].

Bariatric surgery is used for weight reduction in patients with morbid obesity. One systematic review showed that bariatric surgery can improve postoperative conception rates, hirsutism, menstrual irregularities, and hormonal abnormalities in women with PCOS [68]. Another systematic review and meta-analysis about bariatric surgery demonstrated that the incidence of PCOS preoperatively was 45.6%, which significantly decreased to 6.8 and 7.1% at the 1 year follow-up and study endpoint, respectively [69]. Moreover, it also demonstrated nearly a 50% improvement in menstrual irregularity and a 30% improvement in hirsutism [69]. There is still a lack of evidence for the improvement in fertility after bariatric surgery [68, 69]. One report revealed the tendency of increasing infant mortality in the bariatric group and bariatric surgery may have its own unique risk-benefit ratio with regards to pregnancy results [70].

5. Traditional Chinese medicine

Traditional Chinese medicine formulas and herbs have been used to manage the health problems of women for hundreds of years. Classically, Chinese medicine prescription is composed of many herbs to treat a specific disease. According to the principles of TCM syndrome patterns for PCOS, one study showed that Shen deficiency with blood-stasis syndrome was the most frequent pattern noted in these patients, followed by Pi-deficiency with phlegm-dampness syndrome, Pi-Shenyang-deficiency syndrome, and Shen-yin deficiency syndrome [71]. Another study demonstrated that TCM syndrome patterns presented in patients with PCOS were mostly amalgamative, of which Shen deficiency and Gan stagnancy are the basic syndromes [72]. One earlier study revealed that elevated levels of testosterone correlated more with the TCM syndrome pattern of Shen-Yi deficiency compared to other patterns [73]. Interestingly, there is one study that describes the correlation between TCM syndrome patterns of PCOS and ovulation induction effects [74]. The effects of clomiphene on patients with phlegm-dampness accumulation syndrome and Shen-yin deficiency syndrome were poorer than in patients with Shen-yang deficiency syndrome and Gan-stagnancy transformed heat syndrome, which suggested the degree of reproduction endocrine dysfunction or the metabolism disturbance of the former two syndrome patterns were more severe than the latter two syndrome patterns [74].

5.1. Chinese herbal formulas for PCOS

5.1.1. Jia-Wei-Xiao-Yao-San

Jia-Wei-Xiao-Yao-San, also called Dan-Zhi-Xiao-Yao-San, consists of Moutan Radicis Cortex, Radix Paeoniae Rubra, Bupleuri Radix, Angelicae Sinensis Radix, Poria, Glycyrrhizae Radix, Atractylodes Ovatae Rhizoma, Zingiberis Rhizoma Recens, and Menthae Herba. According to the principles of TCM, Jia-Wei-Xiao-Yao-San disperses stagnated liver qi for relief of qi stagnation and suppresses heat and nourishes the blood. One study showed that a danzhi xiaoyao pill could improve ovulation rates and pregnancy rates in anovulation infertility patients with PCOS complicated by IR [75]. It was also reported as the most frequently prescribed formula for patients with PCOS in north Taiwan [76].

5.1.2. Wen-Jing-Tang

Wen-Jing-Tang consists of *Cinnamomi Ramulus, Evodiae Fructus, Ligustici Rhizoma, Angelicae sinensis Radix, Paeoniae Radix, Ginseng Radix, Glycyrrhizae Radix, Zingiberis Rhizoma Recens, Moutan Radicis Cortex, Ophiopogonis Tuber, Pinelliae Tuber,* and *Asini Corii Gelatinum.* According to the principles of TCM, Wen-Jing-Tang would promote blood circulation to dispel blood stasis, dispels cold by warming the meridians, benefits qi, and nourishes the blood. One study showed that Wen-Jing-Tang was effective in regulating endocrine conditions in the treatment of ovulation disorders in patients with PCOS [77]. It suggested that Wen-Jing-Tang is adequate for the clinical management of PCOS in women with various constitutions (as determined by the matching theory of eight-principle pattern identification) [77].

5.1.3. Cang-Fu-Dao-Tan-Wan

Cang-Fu-Dao-Tan-Wan consists of *Atractylodes Lanceae Rhizoma, Cyperi Rhizoma, Pinelliae Rhizoma, Citri Reticulata Pericarpium, Poria, Citrus aurantium L., Glycyrrhiza Radix,* and *Arisaema heterophyllum Bl.* According to principles of TCM, Cang-Fu-Dao-Tan-Wan resolves phlegm and dissipates masses, eliminates dampness, and relieves depression. One study evaluated the efficacy of a modified Cangfu Daotan pill combined with clomiphene in patients with PCOS. The results showed that the modified Cangfu Daotan pill could improve symptoms, increase ovarian artery blood flow, and lower FSH and LH [78]. Another study evaluated a modified Cangfu Daotan Decoction (MCDD) on endometrial receptivity in infertility patients with PCOS [79]. MCDD could increase pregnancy rates with improving insulin resistance, endometrial blood flow, endometrial receptivity, and increasing the uncoupling protein (UCP2) expression [79]. UCP2 expression, negatively regulating the hypersensitivity of insulin, has been reported to be significantly higher in early stage follicles of ovary tissue in PCOS patients [80], but the mechanism and function in the endometrium remains unknown.

5.2. Single Chinese herbs for PCOS

5.2.1. Cyperi Rhizoma

Cyperi Rhizoma, also called Xiang Fu in Chinese, originates from dried roots of *Cyperus rotundus L.* According to the principles of TCM, it can disperse and rectify depressed liver-energy, regulating menstruation, and arresting pain. *Cyperi Rhizoma* was also reported as the most frequently prescribed single herb in north Taiwan for patients with PCOS [76]. It may have potential for PCOS treatment due to its pharmacological benefits resulting in anti-androgenic, anti-diabetic, anti-lipidemic, anti-obesity, and weight-control effects in obese patients according to the present research results [81, 82].

http://dx.doi.org/10.5772/intechopen.71654

5.2.2. Radix Salvia Miltiorrhiza

Radix Salvia Miltiorrhiza, also called Dan Shen in Chinese, originates from dried roots of *Salvia miltiorrhiza Bunge*. According to the principles of TCM, Dan Shen can promote blood flow to regulate menstruation, cool blood, and dispel blood stasis. Tanshinone, the main ingredient of *Salvia miltiorrhiza Bunge* [83], may decrease the level of androgen and improve the index of lipid metabolism, such as lower total cholesterol and TG, and increase HDL levels, in patients with PCOS [84]. Some animal studies have shown that Cryptotanshinone can reverse reproductive disturbances by decreasing the levels of SHBG, testosterone, estradiol, and LH, as well as the LH/FSH ratio, and can improve metabolic disturbances, such as abnormal levels of LDL-C and FINS by dehydroepiandrosterone (DHEA)-induced PCOS [84, 85].

5.2.3. Coptidis Rhizoma

Coptidis Rhizoma, also called Huang Lian in Chinese, originates from dried roots of *Coptis deltoidea C.y.Cheng et Hsiao.* or *Coptis chinensis Franch.* or *Coptis teeta* Wall. According to the principles of TCM, *Coptidis Rhizoma* can clear heat, eliminate dampness, spill fire, and induce detoxification. The isoquinoline alkaloid and the major constituent, berberine, are derived from this herb [86]. A previous randomized study showed that berberine, compared with metformin, could decrease BMI, lipid parameters, and total FSH requirements, and increase the live birth rate with fewer gastrointestinal adverse events in patients with PCOS undergoing IVF treatment [87]. Another earlier randomized study demonstrated that berberine, compared with metformin, could reduce total cholesterol, TG, LDL-C, WC, and waist-to-hip ratio, as well as elevate HDL-C and SHBG in patients with PCOS [88]. *Coptidis Rhizoma* may have potential for the management of PCOS.

6. Acupuncture and moxibustion

As with TCM formulas and single Chinese herbal therapy, acupuncture and moxibustion have also been used to treat clinical manifestations of PCOS for hundreds of years. Traditionally, acupuncture and moxibustion were performed by inserting needles into or burning moxa sticks upon specific points (acupoints) on the meridians of the body surface. Acupuncture and moxibustion work by regulating energy flow, also called Qi in Chinese, over the meridians. Newer therapeutic methods include electro-acupuncture (EA), laser-acupuncture, burning moxa granules on the top of the needle, points pasting, and far-infrared moxibustion.

Clinical effects of acupuncture are mediated by activation of somatic afferent nerves innervating the skin and muscle, which, via modulation of the activity in the somatic and autonomic nervous system, may regulate metabolic and endocrine functions in patients with PCOS [89]. One analysis showed that the acupoints of Sanyinjiao (SP 6), Guanyuan (CV 4), Zigong (EX-CA 1), Zhongji (CV 3), and Qihai (CV 6) are most frequently used in the clinical management of acupuncture for patients with PCOS [90]. This report also demonstrated the meridians of the main acupoints are the conception vessel, stomach meridian of the foot-yangming, and the spleen meridian of foot-taiyin. The main acupoints are distributed in the lower limbs, lower abdomen, and back [90]. In the special points, usage of front-mu points, five-shu points, and back-shu points are more frequently used and the prescription is usually an average of five to seven acupoints [90].

One prospective clinical study investigated responses to 5 weeks of EA in overweight-obese women with PCOS [91]. The results showed that HbA1c levels and circulating and adipose tissue androgens were significantly decreased, together with modulation of vagal activity and adipose tissue sympathetic activity [91]. A systematic review and meta-analysis demonstrated that manual acupuncture (MA) or EA can improve clinical pregnancy rates and ongoing pregnancy rates, and lower the risk of ovarian hyperstimulation syndrome (OHSS) in women with PCOS undergoing in vitro fertilization (IVF) or intracytoplasmic sperm injection (ICSI) [92]. Another RCT revealed that serum androgens decreased and menstrual frequency increased after 16 weeks of EA intervention, while the acne improved after the 16-week follow-up in the EA group compared to the exercise group [93]. The other RCT showed that serum levels of AMH were significantly decreased in the EA group compare with the change in the exercise group after 16 weeks of intervention, but there was no difference in the exercise group and the no intervention group at 32 weeks follow-up [94]. An earlier RCT found that abdominal acupuncture for obese patients with PCOS can reduce BMI and WHR and increase menstrual frequency more effectively, and with fewer adverse effects, than metformin after a 6-month trial [95].

True (EA group) and sham (Park sham device group) acupuncture (EA V.S. Park sham device) may have similar effects on mean ovulation rates and reproductive endocrine changes, but the true acupuncture group could show lower fasting insulin and free testosterone levels after 8 weeks of intervention [96]. Another RCT showed that the utilization of acupuncture with or without clomiphene, compared with control acupuncture and placebo, did not increase live births in patients with PCOS [97]. A recent systematic review and meta-analysis demonstrated that acupuncture may be more likely to improve ovulation rates and menstruation frequency than no acupuncture in patients with PCOS [98]. This report also noted that acupuncture could be as an adjunct to medication with regard to LH, LH/FSH ratio, testosterone, fasting insulin, and pregnancy rates [98]. Another study revealed that there were very few RCTs have been reported and there was deficient evidence to support the use of acupuncture for management of ovulation problems in patients with PCOS [99].

7. Conclusions

Traditional Chinese medicine formulas or single herbs have been shown to be effective in many clinical or animal studies to restore regular menstruation, relieve symptoms, and improve ovulation dysfunction in patients with PCOS. Acupuncture, both EA and MA, have the potential to change the local ovarian hyperandrogenic environment and improve reproductive and endocrine metabolic disorders in PCOS. Thus, better outcomes can be achieved through complementary therapy with TCM for PCOS, expediting and boosting treatment efficacy, and ultimately leading to decreased medical costs. However, more clear, effective, and safe evidence for the use of TCM management for PCOS is needed in the future.

Author details

Yen-Nung Liao[1], Wen-Long Hu[1,2,3] and Yu-Chiang Hung[1,4]*

*Address all correspondence to: hungyuchiang@gmail.com

1 Department of Chinese Medicine, Kaohsiung Chang Gung Memorial Hospital and School of Traditional Chinese Medicine, Chang Gung University College of Medicine, Kaohsiung, Taiwan

2 Fooyin University College of Nursing, Kaohsiung, Taiwan

3 Kaohsiung Medical University College of Medicine, Kaohsiung, Taiwan

4 School of Chinese Medicine for Post Baccalaureate, I-Shou University, Kaohsiung, Taiwan

References

[1] Stein IF, Leventhal ML. Amenorrhea associated with bilateral polycystic ovaries. American Journal of Obstetrics and Gynecol. 1935;**29**:181-191

[2] Sirmans SM, Pate KA. Epidemiology, diagnosis, and management of polycystic ovary syndrome. Clinical Epidemiology. 2013;**6**:1-13. DOI: 10.2147/CLEP.S37559

[3] Szydlarska1 D, Machaj M, Jakimiuk A. History of discovery of polycystic ovary syndrome. Advances in Clinical and Experimental Medicine. 2017;**26**:555-558. DOI: 10.17219/acem/61987

[4] Zawadski JK, Dunaif A. 1992 Diagnostic criteria for polycystic ovary syndrome: Towards a rational approach. In: Dunaif A, Givens JR, Haseltine FP, Merriam GR, eds. Polycystic ovary syndrome. Boston: Blackwell Scientific Publications; p. 377-384

[5] Rotterdam ESHRE/ASRM-Sponsored PCOS Consensus Workshop Group. Revised 2003 consensus on diagnostic criteria and long-term health risks related to polycystic ovary syndrome. Fertility and Sterility. 2004;**81**:19-25. DOI: 10.1016/j.fertnstert.2003.10.004

[6] Azziz R, Carmina E, Dewailly D, Diamanti-Kandarakis E, Escobar-Morreale HF, Futterweit W, Janssen OE, Legro RS, Norman RJ, Taylor AE, Witchel SF. Androgen Excess Society. Positions statement: Criteria for defining polycystic ovary syndrome as a predominantly hyperandrogenic syndrome: An Androgen Excess Society guideline. Journal of Clinical and Endocrinology Metabolism. 2006;**91**:4237-4245. DOI: 10.1210/jc.2006-0178

[7] Lizneva D, Suturina L, Walker W, Brakta S, Gavrilova-Jordan L, Azziz R. Criteria, prevalence, and phenotypes of polycystic ovary syndrome. Fertility and Sterility. 2016;**106**:6-15. DOI: 10.1016/j.fertnstert.2016.05.003

[8] National Institutes of Health. Evidence-based methodology workshop on polycystic ovary syndrome, December 3-5, 2012 [Internet]. Available from: https://prevention.nih.gov/docs/programs/pcos/FinalReport.pdf [Accessed 2017-6-25]

[9] Azziz R, Carmina E, Chen Z, Dunaif A, Laven JS, Legro RS, Lizneva D, Natterson-Horowtiz B, Teede HJ, Yildiz BO. Polycystic ovary syndrome. Natural Reviews Disease Primers. 2016;**2**:16057. DOI: 10.1038/nrdp.2016.57

[10] Wang S, Alvero R. Racial and ethnic differences in physiology and clinical symptoms of polycystic ovary syndrome. Seminars in Reproductive Medicine. 2013;**31**:365-369. DOI: 10.1055/s-0033-1348895

[11] Huang Z, Yong EL. Ethnic differences: Is there an Asian phenotype for polycystic ovarian syndrome? Best Practices and Research Clinical Obstetrics and Gynaecology. 2016;**37**:46-55. DOI: 10.1016/j.bpobgyn.2016.04.001

[12] Lizneva D, Kirubakaran R, Mykhalchenko K, Suturina L, Chernukha G, Diamond MP, Azziz R. Phenotypes and body mass in women with polycystic ovary syndrome identified in referral versus unselected populations: Systematic review and meta-analysis. Fertility and Sterility. 2016;**106**:1510-1520.e2. DOI: 10.1016/j.fertnstert.2016.07.1121

[13] Lim SS, Davies MJ, Norman RJ, Moran LJ. Overweight, obesity and central obesity in women with polycystic ovary syndrome: A systematic review and meta-analysis. Human Reproduction Update. 2012;**18**:618-637. DOI: 10.1093/humupd/dms030

[14] Orio F, Muscogiuri G, Nese C, Palomba S, Savastano S, Tafuri D, Colarieti G, La Sala G, Colao A, Yildiz BO. Obesity, type 2 diabetes mellitus and cardiovascular disease risk: An uptodate in the management of polycystic ovary syndrome. European Journal of Obstetrics and Gynecology and Reproductive Biology. 2016;**207**:214-219. DOI: 10.1016/j.ejogrb.2016.08.026

[15] Cascella T, Palomba S, De Sio I, Manguso F, Giallauria F, De Simone B, Tafuri D, Lombardi G, Colao A, Orio F. Visceral fat is associated with cardiovascular risk in women with polycystic ovary syndrome. Human Reproduction. 2008;**23**:153-159. DOI: 10.1093/humrep/dem356

[16] Randeva HS, Tan BK, Weickert MO, Lois K, Nestler JE, Sattar N, Lehnert H. Cardiometabolic aspects of the polycystic ovary syndrome. Endocrine Reviews. 2012;**33**:812-841. DOI: 10.1210/er.2012-1003

[17] Peppard HR, Marfori J, Iuorno MJ, Nestler JE. Prevalence of polycystic ovary syndrome among premenopausal women with Type 2 diabetes. Diabetes Care. 2001;**24**:1050-1052. PMID: 11375369

[18] Kim JJ, Choi YM. Dyslipidemia in women with polycystic ovary syndrome. Obstetrics and Gynecology Science. 2013;**56**:137-142. DOI: 10.5468/ogs.2013.56.3.137

[19] Legro RS, Kunselman AR, Dunaif A. Prevalence and predictors of dyslipidemia in women with polycystic ovary syndrome. American Journal of Medicine. 2001;**111**:607-613. PMID: 11755503

[20] Wild RA, Rizzo M, Clifton S, Carmina E. Lipid levels in polycystic ovary syndrome: Systematic review and met analysis. Fertility and Sterility. 2011;**95**:1073-1079. DOI: 10.1016/j.fertnstert.2010.12.027

[21] Orbetzova MM, Shigarminova RG, Genchev GG, Milcheva BA, Lozanov LB, Genov NS, Zacharieva SZ. Role of 24-hour monitoring in assessing blood pressure changes in polycystic ovary syndrome. Folia Med (Plovdiv). 2003;**45**:21-25. PMID: 15366662

[22] Baldani DP, Skrgatic L, Ougouag R. Polycystic ovary syndrome: Important underrecognised cardiometabolic risk factor in reproductive-age women. International Journal of Endocrinology. 2015;**2015**:786362. DOI: 10.1155/2015/786362

[23] de Groot PC, Dekkers OM, Romijn JA, Dieben SW, Helmerhorst FM. PCOS, coronary heart disease, stroke and the influence of obesity: A systematic review and meta-analysis. Human Reproduction Update. 2011;**17**:495-500. DOI: 10.1093/humupd/dmr001

[24] Balen AH, Morley LC, Misso M, Franks S, Legro RS, Wijeyaratne CN, Stener-Victorin E, Fauser BC, Norman RJ, Teede H. The management of anovulatory infertility in women with polycystic ovary syndrome: An analysis of the evidence to support the development of global WHO guidance. Human Reproduction Update. 2016;**22**:687-708. DOI: 10.1093/humupd/dmw025

[25] Thessaloniki ESHRE/ASRM-Sponsored PCOS Consensus Workshop Group. Consensus on infertility treatment related to polycystic ovary syndrome. Human Reproduction. 2008;**23**:462-477. DOI: 10.1093/humrep/dem426

[26] Barry JA, Azizia MM, Hardiman PJ. Risk of endometrial, ovarian and breast cancer in women with polycystic ovary syndrome: A systematic review and meta-analysis. Human Reproduction Update. 2014;**20**:748-758. DOI: 10.1093/humupd/dmu012

[27] Paixão L, Ramos RB, Lavarda A, Morsh DM, Spritzer PM. Animal models of hyperandrogenism and ovarian morphology changes as features of polycystic ovary syndrome: A systematic review. Reproductive Biology and Endocrinology. 2017;**15**:12. DOI: 10.1186/s12958-017-0231-z

[28] Dumesic DA, Goodarzi MO, Chazenbalk GD, Abbott DH. Intrauterine environment and polycystic ovary syndrome. Seminars in Reproductive Medicine. 2014;**32**:159-165. DOI: 10.1055/s-0034-1371087

[29] De Leo V, Musacchio MC, Cappelli V, Massaro MG, Morgante G, Petraglia F. Genetic, hormonal and metabolic aspects of PCOS: An update. Reproductive Biology and Endocrinology. 2016;**14**:38. DOI: 10.1186/s12958-016-0173-x

[30] Trofimova T, Lizneva D, Suturina L, Walker W, Chen YH, Azziz R, Layman LC. Genetic basis of eugonadal and hypogonadal female reproductive disorders. Best Practices in Research and Clinical Obstetrics and Gynaecology. 2017; pii: S1521-6934(17)30069-X. DOI: 10.1016/j.bpobgyn.2017.05.003

[31] Jones MR, Goodarzi MO. Genetic determinants of polycystic ovary syndrome: Progress and future directions. Fertility and Sterility. 2016;**106**:25-32. DOI: 10.1016/j.fertnstert.2016.04.040

[32] Barbieri RL, Ehrmann DA. [Internet]. 2017. Available from: https://www.uptodate.com/contents/diagnosis-of-polycystic-ovary-syndrome-in-adults?source=search_result&search=pcos%20diagnosis%20adult&selectedTitle=1~150 [Accessed: 2017-6-30]

[33] Dewailly D. Diagnostic criteria for PCOS: Is there a need for a rethink? Best Practice & Research Clinical Obstetrics & Gynaecology. 2016;**37**:5-11. DOI: 10.1016/j.bpobgyn.2016.03.009

[34] van Hooff MH, Voorhorst FJ, Kaptein MB, Hirasing RA, Koppenaal C, Schoemaker J. Predictive value of menstrual cycle pattern, body mass index, hormone levels and polycystic ovaries at age 15 years for oligo-amenorrhoea at age 18 years. Human Reproduction. 2004;**19**:383-392. DOI: 10.1093/humrep/deh079

[35] Balen A, Conway G, Kaltsas G. Polycystic ovary syndrome: The spectrum of the disorder in 1741 patients. Human Reproduction. 1995;**10**:2107-2111. PMID: 8567849

[36] Hart R. Definitions, prevalence and symptoms of polycystic ovaries and the polycystic ovary syndrome. In: Allahbadia GN, Agrawal R, editors. Polycystic Ovary Syndrome. Kent, UK: Anshan, Ltd; 2007:15-26

[37] Ogden C, Carroll M. Prevalence of Obesity among Children and Adolescents: United States, Trends 1963-1965 through 2007-2008. Hyattsville, MD: Centers for Disease Control and Prevention, National Center for Health Statistics; 2010

[38] Glueck CJ, Aregawi D, Winiarska M, Agloria M, Luo G, Sieve L, Wang P. Metformin-diet ameliorates coronary heart disease risk factors and facilitates resumption of regular menses in adolescents with polycystic ovary syndrome. Journal of Pediatric Endocrinology and Metabolism. 2006;**19**:831-842. PMID: 16886591

[39] Glueck CJ, Morrison JA, Friedman LA, Goldenberg N, Stroop DM, Wang P. Obesity, free testosterone, and cardiovascular risk factors in adolescents with polycystic ovary syndrome and regularly cycling adolescents. Metabolism 2006;**55**:508-514. DOI: 10.1016/j.metabol.2005.11.003

[40] Glueck CJ, Morrison JA, Wang P. Insulin resistance, obesity, hypofibrinolysis, hyperandrogenism, and coronary heart disease risk factors in 25 pre-perimenarchal girls age < or =14 years, 13 with precocious puberty, 23 with a first-degree relative with polycystic ovary syndrome. Journal of Pediatric Endocrinology and Metabolism. 2008;**21**:973-984. PMID: 19209619

[41] Zhu RY, Wong YC, Yong EL. Sonographic evaluation of polycystic ovaries. Best Practice & Research Clinical Obstetrics & Gynaecology. 2016;**37**:25-37. DOI: 10.1016/j.bpobgyn.2016.02.005

[42] Balen AH, Laven JS, Tan SL, Dewailly D. Ultrasound assessment of the polycystic ovary: International consensus definitions. Human Reproduction Update. 2003;**9**:505-514. PMID: 14714587

[43] Dewailly D, Lujan ME, Carmina E, Cedars MI, Laven J, Norman RJ, Escobar-Morreale HF. Definition and significance of polycystic ovarian morphology: A task force report from the androgen excess and polycystic ovary syndrome society. Human Reproduction Update. 2014;**20**:334-352. DOI: 10.1093/humupd/dmt061

[44] Ozzola G. Anti-Müllerian hormone: A brief review of the literature. Clin Ter. 2017;**168**: e14-e22. DOI: 10.7417/CT.2017.1976

[45] Łebkowska A, Kowalska I. Anti-Müllerian hormone and polycystic ovary syndrome. Endokrynologia Polska. 2017;**68**:74-78. DOI: 10.5603/EP.a2016.0065

[46] Tal R, Seifer DB, Khanimov M, Malter HE, Grazi RV, Leader B. Characterization of women with elevated antimüllerian hormone levels (AMH): Correlation of AMH with polycystic ovarian syndrome phenotypes and assisted reproductive technology outcomes. American Journal of Obstetrics & Gynecology. 2014;**211**:59.e1-8. DOI: 10.1016/j.ajog.2014.02.026

[47] Andrade VH, Mata AM, Borges RS, Costa-Silva DR, Martins LM, Ferreira PM, Cunha-Nunes LC, Silva BB. Current aspects of polycystic ovary syndrome: A literature review. Revista Da Associacao Medica Brasileira (1992). 2016;**62**:867-871. DOI: 10.1590/1806-9282.62.09.867

[48] Nayaker BS, Thomas S, Ramachandran S, Loganathan S, Sundari M, Mala K. Polycystic ovarian syndrome-associated cardiovascular complications: An overview of the association between the biochemical markers and potential strategies for their prevention and elimination. Diabetes & Metabolic Syndrome. 2017; pii: S1871-4021(17)30165-0. DOI: 10.1016/j.dsx.2017.07.004

[49] Bates GW, Legro RS. Longterm management of Polycystic Ovarian Syndrome (PCOS). Molecular Cell Endocrinology. 2013;**373**:91-97. DOI: 10.1016/j.mce.2012.10.029

[50] Faghfoori Z, Fazelian S, Shadnoush M, Goodarzi R. Nutritional management in women with polycystic ovary syndrome: A review study. Diabetes & Metabolic Syndrome. 2017; pii: S1871-4021(17)30011-5. DOI: 10.1016/j.dsx.2017.03.030

[51] Harrison CL, Lombard CB, Moran LJ, Teede HJ. Exercise therapy in polycystic ovary syndrome: A systematic review. Human Reproduction Update. 2011;**17**:171-183. DOI: 10.1093/humupd/dmq045

[52] De Sousa SM Dr, Norman RJ Prof. Metabolic syndrome, diet and exercise. Best Practice & Research Clinical Obstetrics & Gynaecology. 2016;**37**:140-151. DOI: 10.1016/j.bpobgyn.2016.01.006

[53] Wild RA, Carmina E, Diamanti-Kandarakis E, Dokras A, Escobar-Morreale HF, Futterweit W, Lobo R, Norman RJ, Talbott E, Dumesic DA. Assessment of cardiovascular risk and prevention of cardiovascular disease in women with the polycystic ovary syndrome: A consensus statement by the Androgen Excess and Polycystic Ovary Syndrome (AE-PCOS) Society. The Journal of Clinical Endocrinology & Metabolism. 2010;**95**:2038-2049. DOI: 10.1210/jc.2009-2724

[54] Rosenzweig JL, Ferrannini E, Grundy SM, Haffner SM, Heine RJ, Horton ES, Kawamori R. Endocrine Society. Primary prevention of cardiovascular disease and type 2 diabetes in patients at metabolic risk: An endocrine society clinical practice guideline. The Journal of Clinical Endocrinology & Metabolism. 2008;**93**:3671-3689. DOI: 10.1210/jc.2008-0222

[55] Naderpoor N, Shorakae S, de Courten B, Misso ML, Moran LJ, Teede HJ. Metformin and lifestyle modification in polycystic ovary syndrome: Systematic review and meta-analysis. Human Reproduction Update. 2015;**21**:560-574. DOI: 10.1093/humupd/dmv025

[56] Alpañés M, Álvarez-Blasco F, Fernández-Durán E, Luque-Ramírez M, Escobar-Morreale HF. Combined oral contraceptives plus spironolactone compared with metformin in women with polycystic ovary syndrome: A one-year randomized clinical trial. European Journal of Endocrinology. 2017;**177**:399-408. DOI: 10.1530/EJE-17-0516

[57] Tagliaferri V, Romualdi D, Immediata V, De Cicco S, Di Florio C, Lanzone A, Guido M. Metformin vs myoinositol: Which is better in obese polycystic ovary syndrome patients? A randomized controlled crossover study. Clinical Endocrinology (Oxf). 2017;**86**:725-730. DOI: 10.1111/cen.13304. Epub 2017 Feb 10

[58] Skalkidou A, Sergentanis TN, Gialamas SP, Georgakis MK, Psaltopoulou T, Trivella M, Siristatidis CS, Evangelou E, Petridou E. Risk of endometrial cancer in women treated with ovary-stimulating drugs for subfertility. Cochrane Database of Systematic Reviews. 2017;**3**:CD010931. DOI: 10.1002/14651858.CD010931.pub2

[59] Scaparrotta A, Chiarelli F, Verrotti A. Potential teratogenic effects of clomiphene citrate. Drug Safety. 2017;**40**:761-769. DOI: 10.1007/s40264-017-0546-x

[60] Goodman NF, Cobin RH, Futterweit W, Glueck JS, Legro RS, Carmina E. American Association of Clinical Endocrinologists (AACE); American College of Endocrinology (ACE); Androgen Excess and PCOS Society (AES). American Association of Clinical Endocrinologists, American College of Endocrinology, and Androgen Excess and PCOS Society Disease State Clinical Review. Guide to the best practices in the evaluation and treatment of polycystic ovary syndrome—part 1. Endocrine Practices. 2015;**21**:1291-1300. DOI: 10.4158/EP15748.DSC

[61] Hsia Y, Dawoud D, Sutcliffe AG, Viner RM, Kinra S, Wong IC. Unlicensed use of metformin in children and adolescents in the UK. British Journal of Clinical Pharmacology. 2012;**73**:135-139. DOI: 10.1111/j.1365-2125.2011.04063.x

[62] Bednarska S, Siejka A. The pathogenesis and treatment of polycystic ovary syndrome: What's new? Advances in Clinical and Experimental Medicine. 2017;**26**:359-367. DOI: 10.17219/acem/59380

[63] Tang T, Glanville J, Hayden CJ, White D, Barth JH, Balen AH. Combined lifestyle modification and metformin in obese patients with polycystic ovary syndrome. A randomized, placebo-controlled, double-blind multicentre study. Human Reproduction. 2006;**21**:80-89. DOI: 10.1093/humrep/dei311

[64] Oppelt PG, Mueller A, Jentsch K, Kronawitter D, Reissmann C, Dittrich R, Beckmann MW, Cupisti S. The effect of metformin treatment for 2 years without caloric restriction on endocrine and metabolic parameters in women with polycystic ovary syndrome. Experimental and Clinical Endocrinology & Diabetes. 2010;**118**:633-637. DOI: 10.1055/s-0029-1237705

[65] Lizneva D, Gavrilova-Jordan L, Walker W, Azziz R. Androgen excess: Investigations and management. Best Practice & Research Clinical Obstetrics & Gynaecology. 2016;**37**:98-118. DOI: 10.1016/j.bpobgyn.2016.05.003

[66] Moreno LE, Bonnell A, Neher JO, Safranek S. Clinical Inquiry: What therapies alleviate symptoms of polycystic ovary syndrome? Journal of Family Practices. 2015;**64**:247-249. PMID: 25973451

[67] Raval AD, Hunter T, Stuckey B, Hart RJ. Statins for women with polycystic ovary syndrome not actively trying to conceive. Cochrane Database Systematic Reviews. 2011;**10**:CD008565. DOI: 10.1002/14651858.CD008565.pub2

[68] Butterworth J, Deguara J, Borg CM. Bariatric surgery, polycystic ovary syndrome, and infertility. Journal of Obesity. 2016;**2016**:1871594. DOI: 10.1155/2016/1871594

[69] Skubleny D, Switzer NJ, Gill RS, Dykstra M, Shi X, Sagle MA, de Gara C, Birch DW, Karmali S. The impact of bariatric surgery on polycystic ovary syndrome: A systematic review and meta-analysis. Obesity Surgery. 2016;**26**:169-176. DOI: 10.1007/s11695-015-1902-5

[70] Legro RS. Ovulation induction in polycystic ovary syndrome: Current options. Best Practice & Research Clinical Obstetrics & Gynaecology. 2016;**37**:152-159. DOI: 10.1016/j.bpobgyn.2016.08.001

[71] Li XB, Lan XY, Ou AH. Distribution of Chinese medicine syndrome patterns and its laws in patients with polycystic ovarian syndrome. Zhongguo Zhong Xi Yi Jie He Za Zhi. 2011;**31**:323-326. PMID: 21485070

[72] Zhang XJ, Gui SQ, Qian QH. Prelimary exploration on Chinese medicine syndrome type distribution in patients with polycystic ovary syndrome. Zhongguo Zhong Xi Yi Jie He Za Zhi. 2010;**30**:689-693. PMID: 20929122

[73] Li XP, Zheng CS, Hong ZJ. Correlation between sex hormone and insulin and various TCM syndrome types in patients with polycystic ovarian syndrome. Zhongguo Zhong Xi Yi Jie He Za Zhi. 2007;**27**:996-998. PMID: 18173145

[74] Zhao H, Wang XE, Zhang T. Correlation between Chinese medicine syndrome types of polycystic ovary syndrome and ovulation induction effect. Zhongguo Zhong Xi Yi Jie He Za Zhi. 2011;**31**:896-898. PMID: 21866657

[75] Liu Y, Mao LH. Effect of danzhi xiaoyao pill on ovulation induction of polycystic ovarian syndrome patients of pathogenic fire derived from stagnation of gan-qi. Zhongguo Zhong Xi Yi Jie He Za Zhi. 2013;**33**:1191-1195. PMID: 24273971

[76] Chen HW, Chiang WJ, Chen CL, et al. Characteristics and Prescription Patterns of Traditional Chinese Medicine in Polycystic Ovary Syndrome. Journal of Chengdu University of TCM. 2015;**38**:120-123. DOI: 10. 13593 /j. cnki. 51-1501 /r. 2015. 04. 120

[77] Ushiroyama T, Hosotani T, Mori K, Yamashita Y, Ikeda A, Ueki M. Effects of switching to wen-jing-tang (unkei-to) from preceding herbal preparations selected by eight-principle pattern identification on endocrinological status and ovulatory induction in women with polycystic ovary syndrome. American Journal of Chinese Medicine. 2006;**34**:177-187. DOI: 10.1142/S0192415X06003746

[78] Hong Y, Sun B. Curative Estimation of Using Modified Cangfu Daotan Pill and Clomiphene in the Treatment of Polycystic Ovarian Syndrome Complicated with Infertility. Journal of Sichuan of Traditional Chinese Medicine. 2016;**34**:90-93

[79] Ding CF, Wang CY, Yang X, Zheng RH, Yan ZZ, Chen WQ. Effect of modified cangfu daotan decoction in improving endometrial receptivity in infertility patients with polycystic ovarian syndrome. Zhongguo Zhong Xi Yi Jie He Za Zhi. 2014;**34**:1297-1301. PMID: 25566617

[80] Liu Y, Jiang H, He LY, Huang WJ, He XY, Xing FQ. Abnormal expression of uncoupling protein-2 correlates with CYP11A1 expression in polycystic ovary syndrome. Reproduction Fertility and Development. 2011;**23**:520-526. DOI: 10.1071/RD10266

[81] Pirzada AM, Ali HH, Naeem M, Latif M, Bukhari AH, Tanveer A. *Cyperus rotundus* L.: Traditional uses, phytochemistry, and pharmacological activities. Journal of Ethnopharmacology. 2015;**174**:540-560. DOI: 10.1016/j.jep.2015.08.012

[82] Lemaure B, Touché A, Zbinden I, Moulin J, Courtois D, Macé K, Darimont C. Administration of Cyperus rotundus tubers extract prevents weight gain in obese Zucker rats. Phytotherapy Research. 2007;**21**:724-730. DOI: 10.1002/ptr.2147

[83] Xia Y, Zhao P, Huang H, Xie Y, Lu R, Dong L. Cryptotanshinone reverses reproductive disturbances in rats with dehydroepiandrosterone-induced polycystic ovary syndrome. American Journal of Translational Research. 2017;**15**(9):2447-2456. PMID: 28559995. PMCID: PMC5446527

[84] Zhang JY, Xue HY, Su J, Zuo YH, Fan XQ, Cheng YQ. Clinical effects of tanshinone on polycystic ovary syndrome patients with hyperandrogenism. Guangxi Medical Journal. 2015;**37**:767-769. DOI: 10. 11675 /j. issn. 0253-4304. 2015. 06. 11

[85] Yu J, Zhai D, Hao L, Zhang D, Bai L, Cai Z, Yu C. Cryptotanshinone Reverses Reproductive and Metabolic Disturbances in PCOS Model Rats via Regulating the Expression of CYP17 and AR. Evidence-Based Complementary and Alternative Medicine. 2014;**2014**:670743. DOI: 10.1155/2014/670743

[86] Ong M, Peng J, Jin X, Qu X. Chinese Herbal Medicine for the Optimal Management of Polycystic Ovary Syndrome. American Journal of Chinese Medicine. 2017;**45**:405-422. DOI: 10.1142/S0192415X17500252

[87] An Y, Sun Z, Zhang Y, Liu B, Guan Y, Lu M. The use of berberine for women with polycystic ovary syndrome undergoing IVF treatment. Clinical Endocrinology (Oxf). 2014;**80**:425-431. DOI: 10.1111/cen.12294

[88] Wei W, Zhao H, Wang A, Sui M, Liang K, Deng H, Ma Y, Zhang Y, Zhang H, Guan Y. A clinical study on the short-term effect of berberine in comparison to metformin on the metabolic characteristics of women with polycystic ovary syndrome. European Journal of Endocrinology. 2012;**166**:99-105. DOI: 10.1530/EJE-11-0616

[89] Raja-Khan N, Stener-Victorin E, Wu X, Legro RS. The physiological basis of complementary and alternative medicines for polycystic ovary syndrome. American Journal of Physiology. Endocrinology and Metabolism. 2011;**301**:E1-E10. DOI: 10.1152/ajpendo.00667.2010

[90] Jin C, Pang R, Xu L, Wu Z, Zhao J. Clinical rules for acupoint selection and prescription composition in treatment of polycystic ovary syndrome with acupuncture. Zhongguo Zhen Jiu. 2015;**35**:625-630. DOI: 10. 13703/j. 0255-2930. 2015. 06. 032

[91] Stener-Victorin E, Maliqueo M, Soligo M, Protto V, Manni L, Jerlhag E, Kokosar M, Sazonova A, Behre CJ, Lind M, Ohlsson C, Højlund K, Benrick A. Changes in HbA1c and circulating and adipose tissue androgen levels in overweight-obese women with polycystic ovary syndrome in response to electroacupuncture. Obesity Science and Practice. 2016;**2**:426-435.DOI: 10.1002/osp4.78

[92] Jo J, Lee YJ. Effectiveness of acupuncture in women with polycystic ovarian syndrome undergoing in vitro fertilisation or intracytoplasmic sperm injection: A systematic review and meta-analysis. Acupuncture in Medicine. 2017;**35**:162-170. DOI: 10.1136/acupmed-2016-011163

[93] Jedel E, Labrie F, Odén A, Holm G, Nilsson L, Janson PO, Lind AK, Ohlsson C, Stener-Victorin E. Impact of electro-acupuncture and physical exercise on hyperandrogenism and oligo/amenorrhea in women with polycystic ovary syndrome: A randomized controlled trial. American Journal of Physiology. Endocrinology and Metabolism. 2011;**300**:E37-45. DOI: 10.1152/ajpendo.00495.2010

[94] Leonhardt H, Hellström M, Gull B, Lind AK, Nilsson L, Janson PO, Stener-Victorin E. Serum anti-Müllerian hormone and ovarian morphology assessed by magnetic resonance imaging in response to acupuncture and exercise in women with polycystic ovary syndrome: secondary analyses of a randomized controlled trial. Acta Obstet Gynecol Scand. 2015;**94**:279-287. DOI: 10.1111/aogs.12571

[95] Zheng YH1, Wang XH, Lai MH, Yao H, Liu H, Ma HX. Effectiveness of abdominal acupuncture for patients with obesity-type polycystic ovary syndrome: A randomized controlled trial. Journal of Alternative Complementary Medicine. 2013;**19**:740-745. DOI: 10.1089/acm.2012.0429

[96] Pastore LM, Williams CD, Jenkins J, Patrie JT. True and sham acupuncture produced similar frequency of ovulation and improved LH to FSH ratios in women with polycystic ovary syndrome. The Journal of Clinical Endocrinology & Metabolism. 2011;**96**:3143-3150. DOI: 10.1210/jc.2011-1126

[97] Wu XK, Stener-Victorin E, Kuang HY, Ma HL, Gao JS, Xie LZ, Hou LH, Hu ZX, Shao XG, Ge J, Zhang JF, Xue HY, Xu XF, Liang RN, Ma HX, Yang HW, Li WL, Huang DM, Sun Y, Hao CF, Du SM, Yang ZW, Wang X, Yan Y, Chen XH, Fu P, Ding CF, Gao YQ, Zhou ZM, Wang CC, Wu TX, Liu JP, Ng EHY, Legro RS, Zhang H; PCOSAct Study Group. Effect of acupuncture and clomiphene in chinese women with polycystic ovary syndrome: A randomized clinical trial. JAMA. 2017;**317**:2502-2514. DOI: 10.1001/jama.2017.7217

[98] Jo J, Lee YJ, Lee H. Acupuncture for polycystic ovarian syndrome: A systematic review and meta-analysis. Medicine (Baltimore). 2017;**96**:e7066. DOI: 10.1097/MD.0000000000007066

[99] Lim CE, Ng RW, Xu K, Cheng NC, Xue CC, Liu JP, Chen N. Acupuncture for polycystic ovarian syndrome. Cochrane Database Systematic Reviews. 2016;**5**:CD007689. DOI: 10.1002/14651858.CD007689.pub3